Culturally Competent Care

Guest Editor

DIANE B. MONSIVAIS, PhD, CRRN

NURSING CLINICS
OF NORTH AMERICA

www.nursing.theclinics.com

Consulting Editor
SUZANNE S. PREVOST, PhD, RN, COI

June 2011 • Volume 46 • Number 2

SAUNDERS an imprint of ELSEVIER, Inc.

W.B. SAUNDERS COMPANY

A Division of Elsevier Inc.

1600 John F. Kennedy Blvd., Suite 1800 • Philadelphia, PA 19103-2899

http://www.theclinics.com

NURSING CLINICS OF NORTH AMERICA Volume 46, Number 2
June 2011 ISSN 0029-6465, ISBN-13: 978-1-4557-0539-9

Editor: Katie Hartner
Developmental Editor: Donald Mumford

Nursing Clinics of North America (ISSN 0029-6465) is published quarterly by Elsevier Inc., 360 Park Avenue South, New York, NY 10010-1710. Months of issue are March, June, September, and December. Periodicals postage paid at New York, NY and additional mailing offices. Subscription price per year is, $135.00 (US individuals), $343.00 (US institutions), $244.00 (international individuals), $419.00 (international institutions), $197.00 (Canadian individuals), $419.00 (Canadian institutions), $74.00 (US students), and $121.00 (international students). To receive student/resident rate, orders must be accompanied by name of affiliated institution, date of term, and the signature of program/residency coordinator on institution letterhead. Orders will be billed at individual rate until proof of status is received. Foreign air speed delivery is included in all *Clinics* subscription prices. All prices are subject to change without notice. **POSTMASTER:** Send address changes to *Nursing Clinics*, Elsevier Health Sciences Division, Subscription Customer Service, 3251 Riverport Lane, Maryland Heights, MO 63043. **Customer Service: Telephone:** 1-800-654-2452 (U.S. and Canada); **1-314-447-8871 (outside U.S. and Canada). Fax:** 1-314-447-8029. **E-mail: journalscustomerservice-usa@elsevier.com** (for print support) and **journalsonlinesupport-usa@elsevier.com** (for online support).

Nursing Clinics of North America is covered in *EMBASE/Excerpta Medica, MEDLINE/PubMed (Index Medicus), Social Sciences Citation Index, Current Contents, ASCA, Cumulative Index to Nursing, RNdex Top 100,* and Allied Health Literature and International Nursing Index (INI).

Printed and bound by CPI Group (UK) Ltd, Croydon, CR0 4YY

Transferred to Digital Print 2011

Contributors

CONSULTING EDITOR

SUZANNE S. PREVOST, PhD, RN, COI
Associate Dean, Practice and Community Engagement, University of Kentucky, Lexington, Kentucky

GUEST EDITOR

DIANE B. MONSIVAIS, PhD, CRRN
Assistant Professor, School of Nursing, The University of Texas at El Paso, El Paso, Texas

AUTHORS

ADRIANA ARCIA, BSN, RN
PhD Student, University of Miami School of Nursing and Health Studies, Coral Gables, Florida

JOSEPH P. DE SANTIS, PhD, ARNP, ACRN
Assistant Professor, University of Miami School of Nursing and Health Studies, Coral Gables, Florida

MARK B. DIGNAN, PhD, MPH
Department of Internal Medicine, University of Kentucky College of Medicine, Lexington, Kentucky

JOAN ENGEBRETSON, DrPH, AHN-BC, RN
Judy Fred Professor in Nursing, Department of Integrated Nursing Care, School of Nursing, The University of Texas Health Science Center-Houston, Houston, Texas

KARINA A. GATTAMORTA, PhD
Research Assistant Professor, University of Miami School of Nursing and Health Studies, Coral Gables, Florida

JENNIFER HATCHER, RN, PhD
College of Nursing, University of Kentucky, Lexington, Kentucky

MELINDA HERMANNS, PhD, RN, BC, CNE
Assistant Professor, College of Nursing and Health Sciences, The University of Texas at Tyler, Tyler, Texas

MARY M. HOKE, PhD, RN, PHCNS-BC
Professor, School of Nursing, New Mexico State University, Las Cruces, New Mexico

CARLEE LEHNA, PhD, APRN-C
The University of Texas School of Nursing at Houston, Houston, Texas; Assistant Professor, University of Louisville School of Nursing, Louisville, Kentucky

MARIA C. MARTINEZ, PhD
Research Affiliate, La Casita Center, Louisville, Kentucky

DIANE B. MONSIVAIS, PhD, CRRN
Assistant Professor, School of Nursing, The University of Texas at El Paso, El Paso, Texas

JOSE J. MONSIVAIS, MD, FACS
Director, Hand and Microsurgery Center of El Paso, El Paso, Texas

GIA T. MUDD, PhD
Assistant Professor, College of Nursing, University of Kentucky, Lexington, Kentucky

LESLIE K. ROBBINS, PhD, RN, PMHNP/CNS-BC
Associate Professor, School of Nursing, The University of Texas at El Paso, El Paso, Texas

KRISTYNIA M. ROBINSON, PhD, FNPbc, RN
Associate Professor, School of Nursing, The University of Texas at El Paso, El Paso, Texas

NANCY SCHOENBERG, PhD
Department of Behavioral Science, University of Kentucky College of Medicine, Lexington, Kentucky

AMBER VERMEESCH, MSN, RN, NP-C
PhD Student, University of Miami School of Nursing and Health Studies, Coral Gables, Florida

LINDA D. WILSON, PhD, MSN, CNS
Professor, MTSU School of Nursing, Middle Tennessee State University, Murfreesboro, Tennessee

Contents

> Medical anthropology provides an excellent resource for nursing research that is relevant to clinical nursing. By expanding the understanding of ethnographic research beyond ethnicity, nurses can conduct research that explores patient's constructions and explanatory models of health and healing and how they make meaning out of chronic conditions and negotiate daily life. These findings can have applicability to culturally competent care at both the organizational or systems level, as well as in the patient/ provider encounter. Individual patient care can be improved by applying ethnographic research findings to build provider expertise and then using a cultural negotiation process for individualized patient care.

> This article incorporates the findings from a predominantly qualitative, mixed-method study examining sibling survivors' experiences of a major childhood burn injury into the clinically relevant continuum model as a means of promoting culturally competent and family-centered care.

> This article reviews the culture of biomedicine and current practices in pain management education, which often merge to create a hostile environment for effective chronic pain care. Areas of cultural tensions in chronic pain frequently involve the struggle to achieve credibility regarding one's complaints of pain (or being believed that the pain is real) and complying with pain medication protocols. The clinically relevant continuum model is presented as a framework allowing providers to approach care from an evidence-based, culturally appropriate (patient centered) perspective that takes into account the highest level of evidence available, provider expertise, and patient preferences and values.

> Findings from a qualitative ethnographic study that examined the experiences of a group of persons with Parkinson disease are presented in

this article. Culturally competent care for persons who share a common illness, such as Parkinson disease, is facilitated when the findings are incorporated into the Clinically Relevant Continuum Model. Use of this model allows providers to evaluate and use appropriate published evidence in addition to provider expertise and patient preferences and values.

This article reports findings from a qualitative study that explored the attitudes and beliefs concerning colorectal cancer (CRC) screening among patients and health care providers in Appalachian Kentucky. Results from 5 focus groups are discussed here: 3 with primary care providers and 2 with patients. Although there are some areas of agreement, there are marked differences between the perceptions of Appalachian health care providers and participants regarding CRC screening. This article compares and contrasts those perceptions and provides suggestions for culturally competent practice and culturally relevant research to improve CRC screening in this vulnerable population.

Acculturation does not inform practice in the acute or primary care setting; nor does it explain ethnic disparities in the recognition and treatment of chronic diseases, particularly chronic pain. As clinicians, it is imperative that we recognize contributing factors, comorbid conditions, and the impact of chronic pain on individuals and families. The purposes of this article are to present evidence that exemplifies the nonsignificant role acculturation plays in expression of pain and function of a predominantly Hispanic population on the United States border; and to identify more meaningful perspectives of culture that may lessen health disparities and improve pain management.

Numerous training and education programs have evolved to address culturally competent health care delivery. This article describes an exemplar educational approach used to teach cultural competency to beginning graduate psychiatric mental health nursing students. Using interactive strategies delivered within the 4 phases of the curriculum, the approach has been shown to facilitate students' ongoing journey to cultural competence. Building on baccalaureate nursing competencies, the course addresses attitudes, knowledge, skills, and cultural humility to strengthen cultural self-assessment, cross-cultural clinical practice expertise, and the use of culturally appropriate research for graduate students.

Gia T. Mudd and Maria C. Martinez

Cardiovascular disease (CVD) and type 2 diabetes (T2D) are leading causes of morbidity and mortality among US Latinas. Family history is increasingly used to determine risk for these chronic, multifactorial diseases and to direct prevention interventions. This article provides a brief review on family history screening for CVD and T2D risk identification and presents the results of a pilot study to translate and evaluate the use of a family history tool for Spanish-speaking Latinas. Implications for the use of family history screening to guide CVD and T2D prevention interventions with Latinas are discussed.

Linda D. Wilson

Specific knowledge of African American communities, culture, and history is crucial to achieving culturally competent care. The unique and complex relationship that belief systems have to health care outcomes must be considered for all patients. This is even more apparent in the connection between religion and health outcomes for African Americans. However, as with all ethnic groups, nothing is absolute. Therefore, one must avoid stereotyping and recognize there are differences within each cultural group.

Joseph P. De Santis, Adriana Arcia, Amber Vermeesch, and Karina A. Gattamorta

Hispanic men who have sex with men (MSM) are at risk for HIV and other sexually transmitted infections related to high-risk sexual behaviors. The aim of this study was to test a model that predicts the sexual behaviors of Hispanic MSM that is based on an epidemiologic framework. The results of this study provide some important new information regarding the predictors of sexual behaviors among Hispanic MSM. The final model suggests that mental health is a significant predictor of sexual behaviors in this sample. Major implications for the development of interventions to address high-risk sexual behaviors highlight the need for health care providers and researchers to be cognizant of the influence of mental health issues on sexual behaviors.

FORTHCOMING ISSUES

September 2011
Patient Education
Stephen D. Krau, PhD, RN, CNE, CT,
Guest Editor

December 2011
Victims of Abuse
Sharon Stark, PhD, RN, APN-C,
Guest Editor

RECENT ISSUES

March 2011
Magnet Environments: Supporting the Retention and Satisfaction of Nurses
Karen S. Hill, RN, DNP, NEA-BC, FACHE,
Guest Editor

December 2010
Mental Health Across the Lifespan
Patricia B. Howard, PhD, RN, CNAA, FAAN,
and Peggy El-Mallakh, PhD, RN,
Guest Editors

September 2010
Palliative Care and End of Life Care
Margaret Mahon, PhD, RN, FAAN,
Guest Editor

THE CLINICS ARE NOW AVAILABLE ONLINE!

Access your subscription at:
www.theclinics.com

Erratum

Refers to:

The Implementation of the UHC/AACN New Graduate Nurse Residency Program in a Community Hospital

By Karen L. Maxwell, MSN, RN-BC

March 2011 Volume 46 Issue 1

In the March 2011 issue of *Nursing Clinics of North America*, an error was made to "The Implementation of the UHC/AACN New Graduate Nurse Residency Program in a Community Hospital." The article should have stated the name of the corresponding author's institution as Saint Joseph's Hospital, Atlanta, Georgia.

We apologize for this oversight.

Nurs Clin N Am 46 (2011) ix
doi:10.1016/j.cnur.2011.02.011
0029-6465/11/$ – see front matter © 2011 Elsevier Inc. All rights reserved.

nursing.theclinics.com

Erratum

Preface

Finding the (Cultural) Clues that Make a Difference in Patient Outcomes

More than 50 years ago, the developing fields of medical anthropology and transcultural nursing laid the foundations for the concept of cultural competence.[1] Our knowledge base has exploded since then; yet, the gap between the definition of culturally competent care and the practical application of culturally competent care is still often a mystery.

Currently, cultural competence is defined as a set of behaviors, attitudes, and skills that enables nurses to work effectively in cross-cultural situations.[2] The specific behaviors, attitudes, and skills needed to create successful outcomes haven't been clearly defined, however. Drevdahl, Canales, and Dorcy[3] reviewed the link between culturally competent interventions and outcomes and found a minimal relationship in the literature. It's as if we have the rough draft of a mystery story, but the clues may not help in creating better outcomes. In order to solve the mystery story of cultural competence, we have to be able to identify the pieces of cultural evidence that are critical to good patient outcomes in a given situation. Early in the process, we followed clues, or evidence, that were focused primarily on the idea of race and ethnicity. As the concept of culture began to expand in scope beyond race and ethnicity, more potential clues became available.

The cultural clues of age, gender, education, socioeconomic status, and an illness itself all were admitted over the years as credible evidence, capable of creating their own cultural milieu. But as with any complex plot, they didn't act in isolation. Agar[4] pointed out that it's the intersection of the differing cultural components that impact a given situation. A chronic illness can intersect with a person of a certain age and socioeconomic status to create a specific set of circumstances. Another person with the same illness, but of a different age and socioeconomic status, may find the intersection creates different circumstances. Conversely, with many chronic illnesses, negotiating living with the condition in society creates a shared culture among the persons and their families, thereby creating a specific cultural subgroup. These shared experiences can hold true regardless of a patient's age, education, or socioeconomic status. The cultural components in any given situation are fluid, shifting, and intersecting (instead of obediently static), increasing the complexity for anyone trying to assess them. Even with an array of cultural assessment models to choose from, it can be difficult to tell exactly how to harness all that fluid, shifting, and intersecting information into successful patient outcomes.

Models are not unlike plot outlines of stories; they can help clarify and focus. The Clinically Relevant Continuum Model[5] holds promise as a way to illustrate culturally important clues. This model combines the classic work of Cross[6] with an EBP model.[7]

The Cross model describes a continuum of the development of cultural competence, which is combined with the evidence-based practice model that requires

Nurs Clin N Am 46 (2011) xi–xiii
doi:10.1016/j.cnur.2011.02.012
0029-6465/11/$ – see front matter © 2011 Elsevier Inc. All rights reserved.

knowledge of the research evidence, provider expertise, and the patient's values, beliefs, and circumstances. These components of evidence-based practice become plot lines in the mystery story, and only by finding the clues to each plot line will we be able to solve the mystery.

PLOT LINE 1

Synthesized evidence, in the form of systematic reviews or Clinical Practice Guidelines, shows the strongest evidence for practice. Strong evidence is by definition reproduoiblo, co it's like having a plot line figured out. We can tell who does what, when they do it, and what the outcome will be. We know which cultural clues are strongest in any given situation and that they will create a similar story in similar situations. Language, or the ability to communicate effectively, is emerging as a very strong culturally based clue to outcomes because language barriers easily hamper care at all levels. When we have synthesized evidence available, it's the plot line we should focus on first.

Often, though, synthesized evidence isn't available, so our next best clues available would be the strongest individual research study available on the topic. Individual research studies are like unfinished plot lines; we know they contribute to the whole story, but we can't be sure of their overall contribution until they are written into the overall story (or the larger body of information). The clues may exert a different influence once they are viewed along side other clues that may be stronger. What individually seemed to be a critical clue, or piece of evidence, suddenly diminishes in importance when placed side by side with the other clues on that topic available in the literature. In contrast, a clue may not seem that significant in one individual study but when compiled with other similar studies, it may become a forceful and strong cultural clue that greatly impacts outcome.

Authors in this issue contribute clues to the plot lines of the larger body of work in their specialty areas. The cultural clues in their research (family histories, beliefs and values, behaviors, or acculturation levels) contribute to a bigger story when they are synthesized with the larger body of information available in that field.

PLOT LINE 2

Provider expertise creates another plot line in the cultural competence story. Not only does expertise include knowledge of research findings at all levels but also includes knowledge of the most effective interpersonal approaches for dealing with challenging patients. Kautz[8] provides a stunning example of provider expertise. His knowledge and experience guide his patient interaction in a rehabilitation setting in a way that won't be found in any clinical practice guideline, and couldn't be taught, yet worked in that situation. Expert clinicians have an internalized knowledge and sense of effective strategies and know when an unconventional approach might be effective.

PLOT LINE 3

The plot line that brings patient and family preferences values and sometimes circumstances into the model is the third plot line. The Cultural Negotiation Model[9] can help the practitioner gather information to assist the patient in making an informed decision and open a discussion if his or her own preferences coincide with best practices. This is the ultimate clinical application, in which the provider, bringing knowledge of the evidence, as well as personal expertise and experience to the encounter, is able to individualize the approach based on an interactive process with the patient and/or family.

SUMMARY

The mystery story of cultural competence will change as primary research is carried out with the proper plot lines in place and is then synthesized with similar primary research to determine which cultural clues create a difference in patient outcomes. It's a story in constant revision, and we have to keep our minds open to the idea that today's strongest cultural clues may quickly be replaced as our body of research evidence grows. The culturally competent provider, then, is one who has the behaviors, attitudes, and skills to incorporate the strongest current cultural clues that create a positive difference in outcomes.

The contributions by the authors in this issue of *Nursing Clinics* are important steps toward the evolution of culturally competent care, and their efforts are very much appreciated.

Diane B. Monsivais, PhD, CRRN
School of Nursing
The University of Texas at El Paso
1101 North Campbell Street
El Paso, TX 79902, USA

E-mail address:
dimonsivais@utep.edu

REFERENCES

1. Culturally Competent Nursing Care modules—introduction curriculum. Available at: https://ccnm.thinkculturalhealth.hhs.gov/Content/Introduction/Introduction6.asp. Accessed February 16, 2011.
2. Office of Minority Health Website "Cultural Competency." Available at: http://minorityhealth.hhs.gov/templates/browse.aspx?lvl=2&lvlID=11. Accessed February 16, 2011.
3. Drevdahl DJ, Canales MK, Dorcy KS. Of goldfish tanks and moonlight tricks. Can cultural competency ameliorate health disparities? Adv Nurs Sci 2008;31(1): 13–27.
4. Agar M. Culture: Can you take it anywhere? Int J Qualitat Meth 2006;5(2). Retrieved June 12, 2007, from http://www.ualberta.ca/~ijqm/english/engframeset.html.
5. Engebretson J, Mahoney J, Carlson E. Cultural competency in the era of evidence-based practice. J Prof Nurs 2008;24(3):172–8.
6. Cross T, Bazron B, Dennis K, et al. Towards a culturally competent system of care, Vol. I. Washington, D.C: Georgetown University Child Development Center, CASSP Technical Assistance Center; 1989.
7. Melnyk B, Fineout-Overholt E. Evidence-based practice in nursing & healthcare. A guide to best practice. 2nd edition. Philadelphia: Lippincott Williams & Wilkins; 2011.
8. Kautz D. Great rehabilitation nurses combine art and science to create magic. Rehab Nurs 2011;36(1):13–5.
9. Engebretson J, Littleton L. Cultural negotiation: a constructivist-based model of nursing practice. Nurs Outlook 2001;49(5):223–30.

Clinically Applied Medical Ethnography: Relevance to Cultural Competence in Patient Care

Joan Engebretson, DrPH, AHN-BC, RN

KEYWORDS

- Culture • Cultural competence • Ethnography
- Cultural negotiation • Interpretive ethnography

Culture refers to the shared beliefs and values that underlie and generate social behavior. Culture is the way people make meaning of their experiences and operate in everyday life and develop social organization. Ethnography implies a study of culture, which is "the acquired knowledge that people use to interpret experience and generate social behavior."[1] Culture is a vital component of health and a major factor in the ethos of health care delivery. Cultural issues are a major factor in health-related behaviors and activities and are implicated in health disparities.[2] Culture is a crucial element in the diagnosis, treatment, and care of patients and "shape health-related beliefs, behaviors, and values."[3] Cultural competence has emerged as an important component of health care delivery. Ethnographic research can enhance two important areas in clinical care: cultural competence and evidence-based practice. This article offers an argument for tailoring ethnographic research to better understand how specific groups of people (often those facing similar medical or health concerns) conceptualize their condition and notions about health that provide meaning to their experience and underlie their behavior.

ETHNOGRAPHIC RESEARCH

Ethnography comes from the discipline of anthropology, which is the study of human-kind, including its history and development as well as culture. Ethnography refers to

No funding support was used for this article.
No conflicts of interest in financial or professional relationships.
Department of Integrated Nursing Care, School of Nursing, University of Texas Health Science Center-Houston, 6901 Bertner #764, Houston, TX 77030, USA
E-mail address: Joan.C.Engebretson@uth.tmc.edu

both a product of a study and the research approach used by cultural anthropologists, some sociologists, and other ethnographers. Ethnography studies the ethos or the values and beliefs of a particular person or group of people. Culture is the way people make meaning of their experiences and operate in everyday life. Ethnographic research has been defined as the study of beliefs, values, and actions of a group and to understand another way of life from the native point of view. This understanding of the native's point of view is what sets ethnography apart from other social research.[4] The native perspective may be represented in the local world, a specific setting in society that is generally different from that of the researcher. This setting may be a local community, village, neighborhood, network, or group that shares a common experience such as a chronic illness.[3–5]

Thus, cultural studies can be local and reflect many groups of people who share an experience or event. These shared beliefs can be both explicit and tacit. Explicit knowledge can be easily conveyed; for example, one can tell a new immigrant to the United Stats that the cultural norm is to drive on the right side of the road or a type of currency. Tacit knowledge is more difficult to convey as it relates to more subtle beliefs or conventions that most people are not overtly aware of (eg, different cultures have tacit rules regarding how close one should stand to another in the checkout line at the grocery store).

Equating ethnographic research only with ethnic groups, particularly ethnic minorities, is a very limited view of this approach to research. Essentializing culture to ethnic groups often leads to dangerous stereotyping, and a failure to recognize the innate complexity of the individual and the dynamic nature of culture.[6] Cultural processes include religious practices, sources of personal and social identity, social relationships, and the embodiment of meaning in psychophysiological reactions.[3] These cultural processes may have substantial variation within an ethnic group, related to age, gender, class, personality, and other shared experiences.

In the nursing literature, ethnography is often equated with qualitative research and frequently contrasted with and differentiated from phenomenology and grounded theory. These distinctions do not reflect the breadth of ethnographic research. Anthropology, along with many of the social sciences, has been influenced by philosophic and academic paradigms and theories. Hence, ethnographic research has multiple approaches including structural, interpretive, and critical perspectives. These approaches provide the various lenses in which to frame the research question, design the investigation, and interpret the data. All of these approaches add to the knowledge base of understanding culture. Ethnographers can use a structural lens and produce products such as taxonomies, typologies, or theories.[1,4] Thus, these studies may use methods very similar to grounded theory.

The interpretive approach, which is often associated with phenomenology philosophy and forms the base for phenomenology research in nursing, represents an important epistemological turn in the social sciences, including anthropology. This perspective in the human disciplines leads to more descriptive accounts recognizing the interpretive nature of both the informants and the researchers.[7,8] This interpretive approach refutes the context-free positivist claim that one can reduce the complex world to objective analysis and moves away from the objective/subjective debate.[9] Many ethnographers have incorporated a hermeneutic phenomenological approach to the study of cultural meanings and practices. Another relevant movement in the social science is the focus on how members of social groups attend to their everyday lives. This approach is exemplified by Schultz in sociology and Garfinkel in anthropology.[10] This has clear relevance to nursing as one studies people's experiences, actions, and cognitive constructions about health.

Ethnographic methods may employ fieldwork, formal and informal interviews, group and individual interviews, and artifact examination. Ethnographers may use both qualitative and quantitative methods and often mixed methods in their investigations.

APPLIED ANTHROPOLOGY OR MEDICAL ANTHROPOLOGY

Within the anthropology discipline there has been a recent move toward applied anthropology. One of the major applications is in medical or clinical anthropology. This application uses and expands anthropology's core concepts in an effort to understand sickness:

how it is understood and directly experienced and acted on by sufferers, their social networks and healers
how health-related beliefs and practices fit within and are shaped by encompassing social and cultural systems and contexts.[11]

Incidentally, the Society for Medical Anthropology is the largest society in the America Anthropological Association.[12]

Medical anthropology addresses the clinical issues of how patients interpret their health experiences and their interaction with the health care system. Baer, Singer, and Susser[13] identified three theoretical perspectives for medical anthropology: (1) critical medical anthropology, (2) medical ecological theory, and (3) cultural interpretive medical theory. Critical medical anthropology is based on critical social theories and investigates the ways power differentials shape social processes in health and medicine.

Medical Ecological Theory

The medical ecological framework situates the work in an ecological framework of microculture to macroculture.[14] Using the concept of adaptation, behavior or biologic changes at the group or individual level that support survival in a given environment are the focus of study. Thus, the individual is situated in a cultural hierarchy that influences and is influenced by the macrosocial, political, and economic culture. This is somewhat similar to the systems hierarchies that are familiar to many nurses.

Interpretive Medical Anthropology or Clinical Medical Anthropology

Clinical interpretive theories focus on the interaction of biology, social practices, and culturally constituted frames of meaning that result in the cognitive construction of clinical realities.[15] Some of the related areas are studies of the biomedical system as a culture, the relationship of health care delivery and health outcomes to the political economic systems, and studies of the culture of communities and organizations. Research on various approaches to health and healing such as use of traditional healers or spiritual healing may be particularly relevant to the nursing profession. Also, studies of providers and patients and their interactions or their understanding of illness and disease, as well as studies of patient's experiences with health and illness, have immediate clinical relevance. Studies that focus on individual patients or patient groups have also been called focused ethnographies.

Kleinman,[16] a leading medical anthropologist with background in both anthropology and medicine, has developed a theoretical framework that situates illness and care in the social and cultural world. The health care system is a broad cultural system of socially organized responses to illness and healing that includes patients and healers. Thus, the health care system is seen as broader than biomedicine and embedded in the historical, social, economic, political, and environmental contests (similar to the ecological perspective). Health care is defined as a "local cultural system composed of three overlapping parts: the popular, professional, and folk sectors."[16] The popular sector is the largest sector and is composed of individuals, family, social networks, and community beliefs and activities. This sector is also the least understood. This is where disease is first encountered, and decisions of what to do and when and who to engage for help are made. The professional sector is composed of the organized academic healing professions. In most societies this is the biomedical system, which includes nurses, psychologists, dentists, and other providers. The folk sector includes sacred and secular healers. In some cultures these may be traditional healers, or in contemporary Western society, they are often classified as complementary or alternative healers. These three sectors interact as patients pass between them. Also, with many facilities now providing integrated care and the media that are available to patients and providers, the exchange of ideas among the sectors is increasing. However, each of these sectors has distinct cognitive constructions or orientations about health and illness.

Kleinman[16] also identified key functions of the system as a whole that are performed by the various sectors. One of these functions is the cognitive construction of the illness experience in which the construction of the professional sector is largely around the disease, contrasted with the popular sector's orientation toward the illness experience. Additional functions are establishing strategies for choosing and evaluating health care alternatives and healing activities and therapeutic outcomes. Another very relevant function is the communicative interactions that are used to manage particular illnesses. In these communicative interactions, differences in the explanatory models are likely to exist among the sectors and subsectors of the health care system. Kleinman[16] distinguished five major questions to understand these explanatory models (EMs): (1) etiology, (2) time and mode of onset of symptoms, (3) pathophysiology, (4) course of sickness and severity, and (5) treatment. These questions in various formats have stimulated research in nursing to understand a patient's explanatory model.[17] Understanding patients' EMs is also important in clinical care.[3] These issues were incorporated and expanded to include a focus on healing and maintaining health in Engebretson's[18] study of the constructions of health and healing of lay healers who used touch therapies. These healers' constructions of health and healing were also compared with those of a group of nurses.[19] Adding the focus on health and healing beyond disease to explanatory models tailors this approach even more toward nursing practice. Keeping the anthropological focus of an ecological model of culture, along with the clinical interpretive perspective of medical anthropology with emphasis on health and healing and application to everyday life, provides a very valuable approach for research aimed at informing nurses to provide better patient care. This is congruent with two elements of contemporary clinical practice: cultural competence and evidence-based practice.

CULTURAL COMPETENCE

Cultural competence has become an important issue in health care delivery in the United States. Escalating ethnic diversity has challenged health care providers to provide quality care. National concerns regarding social justice and health disparities have stimulated more interest in addressing cultural issues. Cultural competence has also been linked to sensitivity to culture, race, ethnicity, gender, and sexual orientation.[20]

Several regulations and standards related to cultural competence have been established. The Cultural and Linguistic Services (CLAS) standards were established by the

Office of Minority Health (OMH) in 2001. These standards contain four mandates that are current federal requirements for all recipients of federal funds, and nine guidelines that are activities are recommended by OMH for adoption as mandates by federal and state accrediting agencies.[21] Three of these guidelines refer to culturally competent care, providing care effective, understandable, and respectful care in a manner compatible with patient's cultural health beliefs and practices and preferred language. These also include efforts to maintain culturally diverse staff and provide ongoing education about culturally appropriate services. The other seven guidelines refer to organizational supports for cultural competence.

Cultural competence has been incorporated in the newest Joint Commission for Accreditation of Health care Organizations (JCAHO).[22] In addition to legal requirements of Title VI, which prohibits discriminatory practices based on language proficiency, a number of regulatory agencies have standards or recommendations that address culture and managed care, including the Agency for Health Research and Quality[23] and the Health Care Resource and Service Administration.[24] These standards and regulations deal with two aspects of application: (1) the organizational structure and assuring diversity in health care delivery personnel and the provision of communication resources for cultural groups, and (2) application of cultural competence in the clinical encounter.

While cultural competence is an important goal, several concerns arise about the definition, meaning, and practicality of implementation. Research about and an effort to educate the health care community about cultural diversity are extremely valuable. Additionally, a corpus of literature and a growing number of studies on various ethnic groups beliefs, values, and practices can enhance clinician's sensitivity to cultural diversity. However, application of this literature to clinical practice has often been problematic on the individual patient level. One of the problems is that culture has often been essentialized to specific ethic groups, particularly minorities. This often leads to dangerous stereotyping,[3] or the information becomes irrelevant in clinical application. While general cultural beliefs are important, individual patient care requires additional understanding of patient's experiences with prevention, illnesses, living with chronic conditions, and their experiences of interacting with the culture of the health care system. The application of medical or clinical anthropology may be important in these aspects of clinical application.

CLINICALLY RELEVANT MODEL OF CULTURAL COMPETENCE

A clinically relevant model of cultural competence was developed that linked the concepts of a cultural competency continuum with well established values in health care delivery and further linked with evidence-based practice.[6] This model is based on a well established cultural continuum model[25] that spans cultural care from destructiveness through proficiency. This model (**Fig. 1**) linked destructiveness with malfeasance, in which overt destructive acts are committed against specific cultural groups. Cultural incapacity can be linked with incompetence, in which nonintentional harmful actions occur because of ignorance, insensitivity, or inappropriate allocation of resources. Many regulations, laws, standards, and educational programs have been established to prevent these. Next on the continuum is cultural blindness, which assumes all patients are alike and assures equality of patient care. This is analogous to standardization, in which many formal and informal structures are in place to assure equal treatment to all. While this level is important to avoid the previous destructive levels, it does not provide the best care for the individual patient. Standardizing care is a way to avoid unethical discrimination and promote the reduction of health

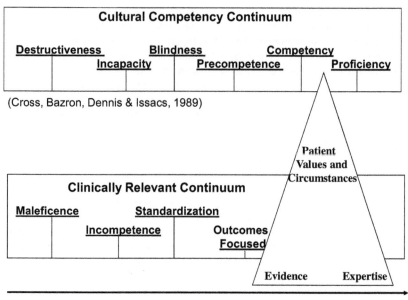

Fig. 1. Cultural competence model. (*From* Engebretson J, Mahoney J, Carlson E. Cultural competency in the era of evidence-based practice. J Prof Nurs 2008;24(3):175; with permission.)

disparities; however, on the clinical level, it can lead to stereotyping, which can be ineffective and possibly harmful.

Precompetence refers to a beginning concern about the access and care of diverse groups of patients (often from specific ethnic groups) and begins to contemplate how groups of people orient around health and health care. This can correspond to a valued goal of health care provision, which is focusing on outcomes and determining patient outcomes such as symptom reduction, adherence to treatment, and patient satisfaction. Cultural competency and proficiency are the highest levels of cultural competence. They define cultural competence as a set of attitudes, behaviors, and polices for an individual, agency, or system that enable effective work in cross-cultural situations. Proficiency involves even higher levels of combining research and influences provision of care and cultural relations. These levels correspond to patient-centered care, in which research and clinical knowledge are applied for individual-based care.

In the model (see **Fig. 1**), an evidence-based practice (EBP) structure is superimposed on the clinical and cultural competence figure. This aligns cultural competence with EBP as defined by Sackett, Strauss, Richardson, Rosenberg, and Hayes,[26] leaders in the EBP movement. They originally defined EBP as a three-legged stool of research evidence, provider clinical expertise, and patient values. In a later edition, Strauss, Richardson, Glasziou, and Haynes[27] added patient circumstances. They noted that all components were required. They reiterated the importance of individualizing the care to the patient and family.

While the bulk of EBP refers to medical treatment based on clinical trials, it is possible that the findings from ethnographic research can add to the evidence base that provides for a better understanding of patient values and circumstances. Findings from ethnographic research related to ethnic beliefs, values, and practices can be extremely valuable in enhancing the policies and organizational protocols and efforts to provide accessible and acceptable care to various populations of patients. This knowledge and understanding also can augment the individual clinician's sensitivity to cultural differences, which can serve to improve communication in patient care.

Application of ethnographic findings related to patients' experiences of daily life with chronic conditions in contemporary society can be applied on both the organizational and the clinical levels. For example, understanding the impact of a patient's condition on the family might lead to routine assessment and providing additional services targeted at the family. Lehna,[28] based on study findings with siblings of severely burned children, advocated for more family centered care to help normalize family function. Often patients and families have developed ways of adapting to chronic conditions that can be shared and used to help other families. Negotiating daily living with a chronic condition is another area of clinical interpretive research. For example, in research with Parkinson disease (PD), patients described many of the issues of negotiating daily activities with the uncertainty of PD symptoms as well as the process of reconstructing their self concept.[29] Patients with end-stage renal disease describe in detail their vigilance to protect their access site during dialysis. This insight may be addressed by providers if they understand how vulnerable these patients feel about their lifeline.[30] A better understanding of this can lead to better anticipatory guidance and more astute assessments of groups of patients who confront managing their condition and still maintaining social roles with families, work, and social interaction in general. The importance of understanding how pain is constructed by various groups is crucial in providing quality care.[31] Getting the accounts of these experiences and how they have attempted to manage this is extremely valuable for clinical practice.

Understanding stigma, which is attached to many disorders, is often based on cultural norms and interpretations of behavior. These interpretations have the potential to impact patient care as well as initiate clinical issues of stress and isolation. Several studies have explored the stigma of mental illness and other chronic conditions. Another issue that is often uncovered in clinical ethnographies is the interaction with the health care system. Morris[32] and Lock and Gordon[33] have discussed the culture of biomedicine as a distinct culture with social roles, modes of dress, unique language, and social expectations. This culture is alien to people outside the health care system and is somewhat akin to traveling to a foreign country. Additionally, this requires a change in social roles when one moves to the patient role. Insights from ethnographic studies that examine culture at the system level can be very valuable to understanding the underlying cultural ethos or how health care systems operate. Understanding how patients navigate daily life with a chronic condition may uncover valuable information for nurses working with these populations. Additionally, research with groups of patients who experience a similar health-related event have the potential to impact the care from both the clinical organizational level as well as for the individual practitioner.

APPLICATION TO THE INDIVIDUAL PATIENT ENCOUNTER

The clinical encounter of individual patient and provider is where expectations of cultural competence are the most demanding.[34] This is an important element of culturally competent/proficient practice. A cultural negotiation model[35] situates the nursing process in the context of the interaction of the individual patient and the nurse. This encounter is situated in the context of the local health care setting and embedded in the ecological context of society, including the health care system and national and global political and economic issues (**Fig. 2**). The nursing process is constructed as an interactive process of cultural negotiation. Kleinman's EMs[3] are embedded in

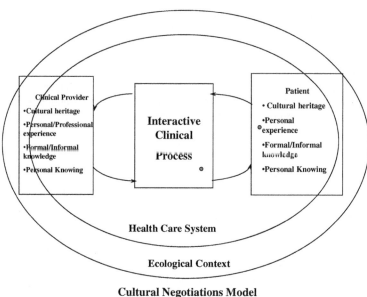

Cultural Negotiations Model

(Engebretson & Littleton, 2001)

Fig. 2. Cultural negotiation model. (*From* Engebretson J, Littleton L. Cultural negotiation: a constructivist-based model of nursing practice. Nurs Outlook 2001;49(5):225; with permission.)

this process, but expanded from a focus on the disease to models of health, illness, and healing to be consistent with the professional telos of nursing.

During this negotiation, the nurse and the patient bring their own cultural heritage to the process. Thus, many ethnic beliefs and values, many of which are tacit, are part of what each enters the negotiation with. It is important here to recognize that the nurse also brings a set of cultural values, so efforts to recognize these are useful and may also enhance awareness and appreciation of how these values influence one's thinking and actions. These beliefs may frame health behaviors regarding food, activity, seeking health care, and the treatment itself. Both the nurse and the patient bring personal experiences to the encounter. For example, the patient may have had past experiences with the health care system or other family members' or friends' experiences with a particular disorder or the health care system. The nurse brings both personal and professional experience with other patients and the health care system. Both bring their formal and informal knowledge to the encounter. The nurse brings formal education, including continuing education, and informal knowledge gleaned from colleagues, reading the literature, and other sources. The client also brings formal knowledge (some may be very well educated in medical issues or have little formal education) as well as informal education. With the advent of computers and electronic information availability, most patients have access to a wide range of information. Some of this information is based in medical sources, while some is not and may be misleading. It is a continuing challenge for providers to assess the patient's information base and sources. Finally, each has a personal knowing or intuitive sense. This is often disregarded in clinical practice. Some patients have a keen sense about their bodies and health, so it is important for a good assessment to acknowledge this.

The process is one of negotiation and interaction and information exchange. The process of assessment is an exchange of expert knowledge, with the patient as expert on him(her)self. The diagnosis is a negotiated process of analysis and interpretation of information. This allows for other issues beyond the medical plan to be clarified and addressed. Planning is joint decision making. With the interaction at this stage, the patient and nurse can determine the priorities and actions needed. Interventions, the next stage, are much more likely to be successful, as they have been mutually derived. a realistic plan of action can then be identified. Finally, plans for evaluating outcomes allow for continued actions and feedback. Knowledge from ethnographic research can enhance the nurse's understanding throughout the entire process.

SUMMARY

Medical anthropology provides an excellent resource for nursing research that is relevant to clinical nursing. By expanding the understanding of ethnographic research beyond ethnicity, nurses can conduct research that explores patient's constructions and explanatory models of health and healing, how they make meaning out of chronic conditions and negotiate daily life. These findings can have applicability to culturally competent care at both the organizational or systems level, as well as in the patient/provider encounter. Individual patient care can be improved by applying ethnographic research findings to build provider expertise and then using a cultural negotiation process for individualized patient care.

REFERENCES

1. Spradley J. The ethnographic interview. Belmont (CA): Wadsworth; 1979.
2. Lillie-Blanton M, Martinez RM, Salagnicoff A. Site of medical care: do racial and ethnic differences persist? Yale J Health Policy Law Ethics 2001;1:1–17.
3. Kleinman A, Benson P. Anthropology in the clinic: the problem of cultural competency and how to fix it. PLoS Med 2006;3(10):1673–6.
4. Spradley J. Participant observation. Belmont (CA): Wadsworth; 1980.
5. Gertz C. Local knowledge. New York: Basic Books; 1983.
6. Engebretson J, Mahoney J, Carlson E. Cultural competency in the era of evidence-based practice. J Prof Nurs 2008;24(3):172–8.
7. Denzin N. Interpretive ethnography: ethnographic practices for the 21st century. Thousand Oaks (CA): Sage; 1997.
8. Denzin N, Lincoln Y. The sage handbook of qualitative research. Thousand Oaks (CA): Sage; 2005.
9. Rabinow P, Sullivan WM. Interpretive social science: a second look. Berkeley (CA): University of California Press; 1988.
10. Holstein, Gubruim. Interpretive practice and social action. In: Denzin NK, Lincoln YS, editors. The Sage Handbook of Qualitative Research. Thousand Oaks (CA): Sage; 2005.
11. Singer M, Baer H. Introducing medical anthropology. New York: AltaMira Press; 2007.
12. Society for Medical Anthropology Website. What is Medical Anthropology? Available at: http://www.medanthro.net/index.html. Accessed December 10, 2010.
13. Baer H, Singer M, Susser I. Medical anthropology and the world System: a critical perspective. Westport (CT): Bergin & Garvey; 1997.
14. McElroy A, Townsend PK. Medical anthropology in ecological perspective. 3rd edition. Boulder (CO): Westview Press; 2008.
15. Good BJ. Medicine, rationality and experience. Cambridge (UK): Cambridge University Press; 1994.

16. Kleinman A. Patients and healers in the context of culture. Berkeley (CA): University of California Press; 1980.
17. McSweeney JC, Allan JD, Mayo K. Exploring the use of explanatory models in nursing research and practice. J Nurs Scholarsh 1997;29(3):243–8.
18. Engebretson J. Urban healers: an experiential description of American healing groups. Qual Health Res 1996;6(4):528–43.
19. Engebretson J. Comparison of nurses and alternative healers. J Nurs Scholarsh 1996;28(2):95–9.
20. Maier-Lorentz MM. Transcultural nursing: its importance for practice. J Cult Divers 2008;15(1):37–43.
21. Office of Minority Health. Public Health Service, United States Department of Health and Human Services. A practical guide for implementing the recommended national standards for culturally and linguistically appropriate services in health care. Available at: http://www.Omhrc.gov. Accessed November 23, 2010.
22. Joint Commission. Advancing effective communication, cultural competence, and patient- and family-centered care: a roadmap for hospitals is a monograph developed by The Joint Commission. Available at: http://www.jointcommission.org/assets/1/6/ARoadmapforHospitalsfinalversion727.pdf. Accessed December 1, 2010.
23. Agency for Healthcare Research and Quality. Cultural competence guides for managed careplans. Available at: http://www.ahcpr.gov. Accessed January 25, 2007.
24. Healthcare Resources and Services Administration. Available at: http://hrsa.gov/OMH/cultural. Accessed November 18, 2010.
25. Cross T, Bazron B, Dennis K, et al. Towards a culturally competent system of care, vol. 1. Washington, DC: Georgetown University, Child Development Center, Child and Adolescent Service System Program Technical Assistance Center; 1989.
26. Sackett D, Strauss SE, Richardson WS, et al. Evidence-based medicine. 2nd edition. London: Churchill-Livingstone; 2000.
27. Straus S, Richardson WS, Glasziou P, et al. Evidence-based medicine. 3rd edition. London: Elsevier; 2005.
28. Lehna C. Sibling experiences after a major burn injury. Pediatr Nurs 2010;35(5):245–52.
29. Hermanns M, Engebretson J. Sailing the stormy seas: the illness experience of persons with Parkinson's disease. Qual Rep 2010;15(2):340–69.
30. Richard C, Engebretson J. Negotiating living with an arteriovenous fistula for hemodialysis. Nephrol Nurs J 2010;37(4):363–74.
31. Monsivais D. Cultural cues: review of qualitative evidence of patient-centered care in patients with nonmalignant chronic pain. Rehabil Nurs, in press.
32. Morris D. Illness and culture in the postmodern age. Berkeley (CA): University of California; 1998.
33. Lock M, Gordon D. Biomedicine examined. Dordrecht (The Netherlands): Kluwer Academic Publishers; 1998.
34. Dreher M, McNaughton N. Cultural competence in nursing: foundation or fallacy? Nurs Outlook 2002;50:181–6.
35. Engebretson J, Littleton L. Cultural negotiation: a constructivist-based model of nursing practice. Nurs Outlook 2001;49(5):223–30.

Families with Burn Injury: Application in the Clinically Relevant Continuum Model

Carlee Lehna, PhD, APRN-C[a,b,*]

KEYWORDS

- Sibling experience • Childhood burn injury
- Culturally competent • Family centered care

The purpose of this article is to discuss how the clinically relevant continuum model (CRCM)[1] and the family-centered care model (FCC)[2] may be applied in the care of sibling survivors of a major childhood burn injury patient as a means of promoting culturally sensitive and family-centered nursing care. The CRCM model proposes that to make cultural competence clinically relevant, concepts from the cultural competence continuum (eg, precompetence, competence, and proficiency) must be linked to accepted values in biomedicine and in the delivery of health care.[1] For practitioners to perform at the minimum acceptable for competent care—using the CRCM, the focused outcomes must use and incorporate the evidence, the expertise of the practitioner, and the patient's values and circumstances.

CLINICALLY RELEVANT CONTINUUM MODEL

A mixed method, qualitative dominant design was implemented. A "case" represented a family unit that comprised one or multiple family members. Participants from 22 cases ($N = 40$ participants) were interviewed in an open-ended question format. In addition, participants were interviewed using the Sibling Relationship Questionnaire-Revised; this was used as a qualitative instrument that allowed for the acquisition of scoring data. One case is presented as an exemplar to illustrate how to facilitate application of findings into the CRCM. The overall thematic pattern for the siblings of children who experienced a major burn injury was that of normalization. Areas of

This research was funded in part by a Shriners Foundation research grant.

The author reports no actual or potential conflict of interest in relation to this article.

[a] University of Texas School of Nursing at Houston, Houston, TX, USA

[b] University of Louisville School of Nursing, 555 South Floyd Street, Louisville, KY 40292, USA

* University of Louisville School of Nursing, 555 South Floyd Street, Louisville, KY 40292.

E-mail address: Carlee.lehna@louisville.edu

doi:10.1016/j.cnur.2011.02.005
nursing.theclinics.com

normalization were found in play and other activities, in school and work, and in family relations with their siblings and their parents. Focusing on returning normalcy to the relationship between the sibling and injured child seems to be the best way of promoting culturally relevant and family-centered care that fits into the CRCM.

FAMILY-CENTERED CARE

For a family caring for a child with a chronic illness, especially a life-altering one, such as a childhood major burn injury, concurrent relevant model is that of providing FCC.[2] The term, FCC, recognizes that the majority of patients have a connection to family supports and networks. It becomes important to link with and promote these existing systems. In this way, family members become allies in enhancing safety and promoting continuity of care. The FCC model encourages family presence and collaboration. Within the FCC model, four concepts are central: (1) respect and dignity, (2) information sharing, (3) participation, and (4) collaboration. When health care providers provide respect and provide dignity, they listen for, ask about, and honor the child's and family's health care choices. Knowledge about values, beliefs, and cultural backgrounds are integrated into the planning and implementing of care, which is also important in the CRCM. Information sharing involves two-way communications between child/caregiver unit and health care provider, which are unbiased, timely, accurate, and useful. For participation, child and family members are encouraged to be involved in care and decision making at whatever level they choose. The final concept of collaboration includes the family in policy and program changes within the health care facility, in professional education, and in health care delivery.

Nurses value both the CRCM and the FCC models because they are collaborative in nature and respectful of the patient's and family's values, beliefs, and ethnic heritage. These models focus on open communication that is nonhierarchal and assists the family unit in decision making, recognizing their expert knowledge about the care of their child having a chronic illness. Implementation of these models differs between individual nurses, by institution, and according to a variety of differing policies.

SIBLING EXPERIENCES AFTER A MAJOR CHILDHOOD BURN INJURY STUDY

An overview of this mixed-method study[3] is described and then a case exemplar illustrates how both the CRCM and FCC model may be used to support standards of care[4] for long-term care in survivors of a major childhood burn injury. Preliminary work in concept explication may be found in earlier work by the author[5] and a fuller study description, including a review of the literature, study methods, and findings, is detailed in recent article by the author.[6]

The design of this mixed-method study was predominantly qualitative, using the life story narrative interview as described by Atkinson[7]; additionally, the Sibling Relationship Questionnaire-Revised[8] was employed as an interview guide and to provide quantitative instrument data. The University of Texas Health Science Center at Houston Institutional Review Board approved the study. Parents or guardians were contacted in the plastic surgery clinic by their care manager regarding study participation. Inclusion criteria were that the burned child was a minimum of 2 years postinjury; the nonburned sibling was present in the home prior, during, and after the burn injury; and the sibling was cognitively intact. Parents or guardians signed consent forms, and the siblings signed either assent forms or consent forms. Interview questions were designed as both open-ended and probe questions, as suggested by Spradley.[9]

There were 40 study participants from 22 families, ranging in age from 9 years to over 30 years, and including injured children, noninjured siblings, and parents. Nineteen participants from 11 families were interviewed more than once. All transcripts were used in the analysis. First, participant-by-participant analysis occurred, then by-family analysis, and finally across-family analysis.[10] As suggested by Aktinson[7] and Miles and Huberman,[10] analysis started at the beginning of the study, with responses grouped according to the injury longitudinal time line (before the injury, at the time of injury, and after the injury) and by family cases. Debriefing occurred between the author and senior researcher. Journaling or use of a field work diary was used to record additional observations, researcher experiences, and ideas or problems from interview sessions.[9,10] Each entry was dated and then reread at a later time. This allowed the author to take into account personal biases and feelings as they related to this study and also the journal was used as an important data source.

FINDINGS

The overall theme for siblings of a child experiencing a major burn injury was that of normalization (ie, creating a relationship that minimized the consequences of the chronic injury). The areas of normalization mentioned were play and activities, school and work, and family relations. Another prominent theme was the process of adjustment, which varied according to many factors (eg, school and community reentry and other life-altering events).

Case Exemplar

This exemplar uses verbatim narratives from a child with a burn injury, his male sibling, and their mother. At the time of the interview, the boys were 16 and 20 years old, respectively; it was 9 years after a moderate gasoline burn injury (30%–59% total body surface area affected). At the time of the first interview, the child with the burn injury was in a plastic surgery clinic for surgical pre-evaluation, just after school was out for the summer. The mother and the adolescent with the injury were interviewed and tape-recorded separately in private rooms near the clinic. The brother was interviewed via telephone. A second interview was recorded 2 years later with all three participants.

The day I got burned (from the child with the burn injury's perspective)...I was in my real dad's foundry (boy at age 7). I was in the attic—sticking gas and lighting it on fire. I caught my arm on fire, started jumping around, and I fell through the roof. I ran outside into the front. My dad picked me up and took me to the shower, laid me on the bed, and my next-door neighbor stuck a towel on my face.

For burn care...I went to Parkland in Dallas. My brother (age 11) was at the house but he wasn't with me at the hospital. My brother visited, I think, on his birthday. My brother stayed with my grandparents. I was there (at the hospital) three months. My mom and my dad were with me. What I remember is...I'd take baths and they (the nurses) would scrub my skin. I had skin grafts so they stuck a cloth on me and everyday they'd have to pull a little bit off. There was pain. I went to rehabilitation near home.

After the burn...teasing...I really didn't get teased until I was in third grade and then after the sixth grade I didn't get teased anymore because I was in football and I started getting stronger. Then, I'd get in a lot of fights, get in trouble, and since I got bigger and stronger, they just got used to me and didn't make fun.

Now (aged 16)…I have girlfriends but I can't call them because I'm grounded. In school, I'm making 80-85, or something like that. In math, I'm making like an 89. Last year, I wasn't a good student because I played football, soccer, and track and ran cross-country. This year, I'm not playing any sports so I can pass my classes. I have to get a job. Last year, I worked at Kroger's and Little Caesar's, too. I want to work at an auto body shop. When I graduate I want to own an auto body shop.

Mom added…Well, their dad passed away, we were home a week and their dad had a brain aneurysm. They just loved and missed him so much. I have a photograph of the first night that we were home with them and their faces are just all lit up. They are just all happy and excited that everybody's back home. Now we have a new dad, we remarried so we all moved down here to be near the hospital for all the surgeries and rehabilitation (Galveston, Texas). He had a moderate burn injury, almost fifty percent of his body was burned. We've been here 8 or 9 years.

My son who was burned has two biologic brothers, one stepbrother, and a half-brother. At the time of the burn injury it was just the three brothers. They were two years apart—they just always play with each other. They played out in the sand pile a lot together. But they fought—they were healthy. The oldest one had quite a bit of school problems while were away at Parkland in Dallas—fighting and that type of stuff. He was the oldest, at age 11, when his brother was burned. Today, they're still the same always playing with each other.

STANDARDS OF CARE

The American Burn Association has guidelines for the operation of burn centers that include burn center verification criteria.[4] Eight prescriptions for services are described in these criteria for the continuity of care program. These criteria should also be interpreted as being standards of care that are expected in all centers providing care to children and adults with burn injuries. These criteria prescribe that the burn center must provide the following services:

1. Recreational therapy for children cared for in the unit.
2. Patient and family education in rehabilitation programs.
3. *Support for family members or other significant persons.*
4. Coordinated discharge planning.
5. *Follow-up after hospital discharge.*
6. *Access to community resources.*
7. *Evaluation of the patient's physical, psychological, developmental, and vocational status.*
8. Planning for future rehabilitative and reconstructive needs.

Four of the eight criteria (those italicized) are supported in the CRCM and FCC models. These involve support of the family, not just the child with the injury; support for the family involves recognizing values and beliefs to facilitate FCC. Follow-up and access to community resources involve creating links for the continuity of rehabilitation between the specialty burn unit and the community. Evaluation of the whole individual involves examining family resources and includes more than just physical needs.

Although the interdisciplinary burn team at Shriners Hospitals for Children Galveston for Children (Galveston, Texas) meets weekly to discuss all their hospitalized children's cases (acute and reconstructive) that week, patients and families are not a part of this conference. Although physicians may obtain patient/family input at the time of their initial assessment, the patient/family dialog needs to be encouraged at all stages of a child's care. Family members need to be supported in undertaking as much of the care and decision making for their family member as they want and are able to perform. Generally, the plan of care focuses on the needs of the child; this needs to be expanded to include siblings at home who are frequently neglected. Follow-up should involve the family as a whole, not just the child with the burn injury, and involves recognizing which cultural practices are supported in the family (eg, father works and mother stays home or single parent family and older girl sibling cares for younger siblings after school and makes dinner).

BARRIERS AND SOLUTIONS FOR PROVIDING CULTURALLY COMPETENT AND FAMILY-CENTERED CARE

The main barriers to providing care reflecting the CRCM and FCC models are the lack of knowledge of main principles of each model (CRCM & FCC); lack of institutional support; lack of adherence to the principles by the health care team; and an individual's personal belief system, which may be in conflict with these models' principles.

Lack of knowledge, a significant barrier to promoting models' compliance, may be overcome through introduction of the CRCM and the FCC model at hospital administrative meetings, at unit staff meetings, and through continuing education offerings. Managers can support staff implementation with monthly recognition by posting pictures or names of the employees who best applied the model in providing patient care in the previous month. Increased use of these models' principles might be tied to unit and hospital satisfaction scores as well. For the case example, including all family members, not only the parents at the bedside, would have been helpful to the family unit. Siblings can be invited to special programs, just for them. Parents can be given educational DVDs to play at home for those family members not at the hospital (eg, siblings, aunts, uncles, and grandparents). Increasing the two-way communication between those at the hospital and those at home may be supported through computers, phones, and other Web-based communication tools for families.

Promoting institutional support for CRCM and FCC principles may be linked to decreasing length of stay, reducing errors, and improving safety through having families advocating for their ill child because of their increased involvement in their child's care. At monthly hospital management meetings, administrators can review pertinent statistics that examine lengths of stay in relation to patient acuity status. Additionally, patient satisfaction scores and individual family comments can be examined to support system-wide changes. Any safety issues should be examined from the system perspective versus assigning blame. Again, nursing administrators may communicate this information to staff in monthly unit meetings.

Lack of adherence to principles may be decreased or prevented when nurses and other interdisciplinary team members (eg, physicians, therapists, care managers, and psychologists) on a burn unit recognize that although they are the experts in burn care, they need to be working in respectful collaboration with the family to promote cure and rehabilitation. This is best implemented by supporting the idea that the family knows their child best and by helping the family gain control after a life-altering change. Family Centered Care with a focus on integrating culturally relevant principles needs to be a primary team goal. It is vital for families to be involved in procedures, daily care (including wound care), care conferences, and planning for discharge to facilitate school and community reentry.

Individuals' personal belief systems, the final barrier, may be explored by staff in group meetings (by unit or hospital-wide across disciplines). Another exercise is for staff to describe the values and beliefs of patients and their families who were or currently are hospitalized. Listing both the staff's and the patients' values and beliefs on paper or blackboards to examine them for similarities and differences would facilitate providing care that is culturally congruent and nonjudgmental.

In the case illustration provided, this full analysis[6] indicated that this family appeared to be a nuclear family with family support in their hometown. There were no differences noted in the values, beliefs, ethnicity, or race between the staff caregivers and the patient/family. If the family had been from Mexico and unable to read, write, or speak English, however, more barriers would have existed for the staff caregivers. Another difference would have occurred if the child's burn injury had been caused by a family member's neglect or abuse. In cases such as that, nurses or burn care team members must remain professional but be advocates for the child by documenting what they see and hear accurately and not supporting the child's discharge to an unsafe environment.

USE OF THE EVIDENCE TO PROVIDE CULTURALLY COMPETENT AND FAMILY-CENTERED CARE

The main thematic finding from this study was that of normalization of the environment in play and activities, work and school, and family relations that may be supported by implementing a culturally congruent and FCC model with families. Evidence from the author's previous study[5,6] in the care of children with a life-altering burn injury suggests that caregivers should encourage developmental play, art, and music therapies in healing while fostering open communication between the health professionals and family members. An injured child should be expected to do school work while in the hospital setting but also should receive assistance from hospital professionals in the transition back into the community and school through the use of videos and visits to the school in the home location. Rehabilitation should be started early during hospitalization with goals set for discharge. Continuity between the hospital and home must be supported for many years, because the child must return for reconstructive surgery many times.

Where changes need to be considered is in having parents/families involved at the same level as a professional in goal setting and achievement. Paramount to attaining normalization is encouraging and facilitating visits via phone, via video conferencing, or in person by siblings and other family members. Supporting parents' disciplining and expectations for their child with burn injury to go to school—and study, pass, and graduate; to have chores at home; and to work are important in normalization. In the case exemplar, the child's burn injury was one of several life-altering events for this family's adjustment. As a part of the yearly reoccurring hospitalizations for reconstructive plastic surgery, these other life-altering events should have been assessed and taken into account in the child's care.

FUTURE RESEARCH DIRECTION/SUMMARY

Findings from this mixed-method study may easily be incorporated into a culturally congruent model and the FCC model. Future research can examine outcome measures evaluating changes in patient lengths of stay, communication between family members at home and those in the hospital, patient/family satisfaction scores, and decreases in patient-care errors, as just a few examples. Research appraising the efficacy and success of the two models should also involve participation and evaluation by siblings and their families.

REFERENCES

1. Engebretson J, Mahoney J, Carlson ED. Cultural competence in the era of evidence-based practice. J Prof Nurs 2008;24:172–8.
2. Institute for Patient- and Family-Centered Care. Frequently asked questions. Available at: http://ipfcc.org/faq.html. Accessed November 1, 2010.
3. Creswell JW, Plano-Clark VL. Mixed methods research. Thousand Oaks (CA): Sage; 2007.
4. American Burn Association, American College of Surgeons. Guidelines for the operation of burn centers. J Burn Care Res 2007;28:134–41.
5. Lehna C. "Sibling Closeness," a concept explication using the hybrid model in sibling experiencing a major burn injury. South Online J Nurs Res 2009;9:4. Available at: http://snrs.org/publications/SOJNR_articles2/Vol09Num04Art07.html. Accessed March 3, 2011.
6. Lehna C. Sibling experiences after a major childhood burn injury. Pediatr Nurs 2010;36:245–51 [quiz: 52].
7. Atkinson R. The life story interview. Thousand Oaks (CA): Sage; 1998.
8. Furman W, Buhrmester D. Children's perceptions of the qualities of sibling relationships. Child Dev 1985;56:448–61.
9. Spradley JP. The ethnographic interview. Forth Worth (TX): Harcourt Brace Jovanovich College Publishers; 1979.
10. Miles MB, Huberman AM. Qualitative data analysis. Thousand Oaks (CA): Sage; 1994.

Promoting Culturally Competent Chronic Pain Management Using the Clinically Relevant Continuum Model

Diane B. Monsivais, PhD, CRRN

KEYWORDS

• Chronic pain • Cultural competence • Pain management

The culture of biomedicine, coupled with suboptimal provider education about chronic pain management, often merge to create a hostile environment for effective chronic pain care. This article first presents a review of the culture of biomedicine and provider education in pain management. Examples are then used to illustrate how the clinically relevant continuum model can be used to assist an individual practitioner in delivering culturally appropriate (patient-centered) care.

THE CULTURE OF BIOMEDICINE

Biomedicine, with its foundation in scientific reasoning, is a system in which objective, measurable data are the standards of communication. Because illness is defined by microbes, toxins, and internal malfunctions,[1(p5)] providers expect objective evidence of an injury or disease to be present if the patient claims to have pain. This idea is strongly entrenched in the health care system as a social system.[2] Consequently, effective chronic pain care is often thwarted by the biomedical culture.

The patient living with a chronic pain condition usually cannot be easily defined and objectified, and proper chronic pain care clashes with biomedicine, as it involves incorporating the patient's subjective experience into a program of holistic care. Biomedicine tends to discount the subjective experience of the patient. Kleinman states "the doctor is expected to decode the untrustworthy story of *illness as*

The author has nothing to disclose.

School of Nursing, The University of Texas at El Paso, 1101 North Campbell Street, El Paso, TX 79902, USA

E-mail address: dimonsivais@utep.edu

experience for the evidence of that which is considered authentic, disease as biological pathology."[3(p32)]

If no observable evidence is apparent (which is often the case with chronic pain), patients have difficulty being taken seriously in the health care system and in being considered a legitimate patient.[4–7] In part, this delegitimization stems from the lack of a diagnostic label. Once a diagnosis is made, there is often a sense of relief because the diagnosis provides a sense of legitimacy, and the patient regains a sense of self. Tait and Chibnall[8] used a factorial design to examine the interaction of medical evidence and pain intensity and found that if supporting biomedical evidence was not present, physicians tended to rate pain and disability lower. In addition to feeling delegitimized by the system, a patient who lacks a diagnosis may also develop mistrust in the physician and the health care system.[9,10] The mistrust arises because the physician is neither able to label the patient's problem nor provide any type of helpful interventions. Because the patient knows the problem is real, the physician's inability to understand and communicate to the patient that there is a problem at all may cause the patient to question whether the provider is competent.

For health care providers, recognition of the key aspects of self-organization (also termed successful coping) in chronic pain provides a useful framework for helping patients achieve successful outcomes. Attributes of self-organization in chronic pain include being believed, accessing credible resources, and taking action and responsibility for one's own rehabilitation.[11]

PAIN EDUCATION OF PROVIDERS

Research on pain management education indicates that it is seriously lacking in curricula for health care providers. Among a sample of 186 family physicians, 60% felt their formal education did not prepare them to manage pain patients and reported frustration in caring for patients in pain.[12] Only 34% of 572 providers in another study felt comfortable in caring for chronic pain patients, with the highest comfort level reported by those who received intensive education after entry into practice.[13] In a national survey, Weiner and colleagues[14] identified numerous areas of pain management that were not being adequately addressed in geriatric medicine fellowship training programs. Tarzian and Hoffmann[15] identified some of the barriers to pain management that nursing home residents face, including providers' personal attitudes (such as fear of addiction) and providers' inability to choose the most appropriate analgesic.

A review of qualitative studies focusing on beliefs about chronic musculoskeletal pain suggests that practitioners may use a biomedical model not because they believe that it is the best one, but because they simply do not know any other method of management.[16] Even though the majority of studies focused on physician education, nurses are often engulfed in the dominant biomedical model as well.

A 2010 review by Breuer and colleagues[17] showed great variation among providers who treat chronic pain, such as primary care providers and pain specialists. Of the groups studied, primary care providers saw the greatest number of chronic pain patients. Unfortunately, they were also least likely to feel confident about their ability to manage musculoskeletal and neuropathic pain.

SUMMARY OF PROBLEMS

Treatment of chronic pain reflects glaring problems for patients and providers on a global basis. Lack of visible pathology can create a sense of being delegitimized and stigmatized for patients when providers do not believe the pain is real. After diagnosis, the mind-body dichotomy produced by the medical model may lead providers and patients to attribute either a physical or psychological cause to the pain problem. The educational system of medicine perpetuates the problem. Pain management education is underaddressed, and societal opioid-phobia and fear of regulatory scrutiny permeates the culture of medicine.

EXAMPLES OF PATIENTS WITH CHRONIC PAIN IN THE HEALTH CARE SYSTEM

The following examples are taken from a parent study that used an ethnographic approach to understand the cultural constructions of chronic pain held by Mexican American women 18 years of age and older living in the El Paso, Texas area. Patients were recruited from a pain management clinic and a fibromyalgia support group to provide information-rich cases for in-depth interviews.[18] Cultural constructions are ways that a group of people organize an understanding about a shared experience.[19] For this article, the cultural constructions surrounding the shared experience of chronic pain within the health care system are presented. The meanings created by these cultural constructions could inform practitioners of areas of special concern or areas of cultural tension, created when patients with chronic pain interact with the health care system.

Many issues were shared by participants, and specific de-identified cases are used for illustration. Mrs K shares many attributes with other study participants. She is 64 years old, receives care from a family physician, and has a 25-year history of back and shoulder pain. Mrs K's back pain reportedly began during her first pregnancy, and was later exacerbated by a fall. She says the pain increased about 10 years ago, and she went to a "back specialist" and a "bone specialist." However, neither specialist was able to find anything more specific than mild arthritis. Mrs K has also been to a chiropractor and a physical therapist, but she states they were not helpful. Mrs K states that she did her own research on the Internet, and based on what she found out about sciatic nerve pain, she believes that is what she has. While interested in being further evaluated, she does not know who would be appropriate to take care of that condition. Because cost is also a worry for her, she prefers to wait until she is 65 (when her Medicare will be activated) before seeing other physicians. She takes medications only when she knows she will be active—such as walking at the mall, cleaning her house, or dancing. She says she does not let her adult children know when she is uncomfortable because she does not want to worry them. Although she is very active, occasionally her pain becomes so severe she must remove herself from family activities so she can rest. She finds this disruptive to her life, and would like to gain more control over the painful syndrome she has.

Just as Mrs K did, many of the participants in the parent study found interactions with health care providers to be frustrating; they expressed the painful symptoms to health care providers, but unfortunately this was often a delegitimizing process.

They don't understand. They just want to do what they think…it is. We are not like cars, they treat us like cars, but we are not cars. It would be easy for us to be like cars–we would say "hey I need this part, take this off and put this on." But it is serious. They need to listen to what the patient is telling them.

Another participant told of a physical therapist who said "It can't hurt that bad, you weren't that injured." A physician asked outright if one participant was faking to receive benefits. The delegitimizing nature of the encounters and frustrations in trying to get help in an unsupportive system caused one participant to say, "If I just damage myself [with a physical injury] it would be better so that way I know exactly what it is rather than, he is looking at me like what are you talking about?" And, on being given a diagnosis of lupus (even though it turned out to be incorrect) the participant said, "But I was thankful, I was grateful that I was sick because I felt that somebody had a voodoo doll on me so I took it as a relief, that I was really sick and I was not imagining." Participants often did not receive necessary care because the condition was not recognized since it was not visible. Health care providers often share the same social and cultural constructions of invisible conditions as their patients.

Although appropriate medication is an important part of the pain treatment plan, in the parent study, societal misconceptions and stigmas regarding medications often blended with individual bias to create a hostile environment for those who needed to take pain medication to control their pain. Patients often simply did not take the medication prescribed because they did not associate themselves with the type of people whom they perceived as needing pain medication (the elderly or drug addicts).

In addition to difficult experiences in the health care system, study participants also gave examples of positive, legitimizing experiences. Finding a specialist who understood how to treat the problem, being listened to, and finding a support group or helpful information all decreased stress. Those who were receiving proper pain management emphasized how important it was to get a proper referral early.

One participant lamented the fact that she had not sought specialty care sooner. "If I would have known that there was doctors that really care about their patients, I would have gone with a specialist at the beginning. We don't go to the doctor so by the time we go, it's too late because the disease has taken the best of the body." Others echoed this sentiment, but stated they were not aware of how to access specialty care.

For women in the parent study, rehabilitation from chronic pain was facilitated when they were recognized as having a "real" condition, and when they were in a setting where best practice pain management protocols were used.

WORKING TOWARD SOLUTIONS

The clinically relevant continuum model (CRCM)[20] provides a useful framework for incorporating both high-level evidence (such as clinical practice guidelines) and lower-level findings (such as individual-study ethnographic research findings) into care. The CRCM links both well-established concepts of cultural competency[21] and evidence-based practice (**Fig. 1**).

Clinical practice guidelines would be equated with standardization on the continuum. For example, pain management guidelines (such as those published by the Registered Nurses Association of Ontario [RNAO])[22] provide only broad suggestions for the provider, and must be used in conjunction with individual patient data for patient-centered care to occur.

The "Outcomes Focused" area of the continuum (see **Fig. 1**) would include standard outcomes of measures such as pain interference with activities of daily living, mobility, overall functioning, mood, depression, and vitality. These measures may serve as a starting point for discussion, but do not generally capture details of individual patient beliefs and values, which are often the determining factor in whether patients have a successful treatment outcome.

The next portion of the continuum brings the evidence-based practice model into play. Patient beliefs and values become an important component under the heading of "Patient Preferences and Values." The cultural negotiation model of Engebretson and Littleton[2] can be used to bring out patient preferences and values, and to arrive at mutually derived plans. In contrast to the traditional model of nursing assessment,

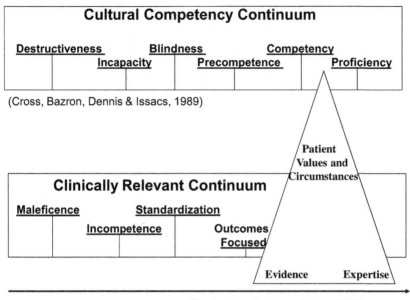

Fig. 1. Clinically relevant continuum model. (*From* Engebretson J, Mahoney J, Carlson E. Cultural competency in the era of evidence-based practice. J Prof Nurs 2008;24(3):175; with permission.)

diagnosis, planning, and intervention, which is a provider-driven process, the negotiation model views the patient as providing expert knowledge of his own condition. While the provider brings knowledge from research evidence and a clinical background, the patient provides specifics about his or her own situation, and joint decision making and planning can occur.

The provider is able to move toward cultural competency when information gathered while using the cultural negotiation model is incorporated into the CRCM. For example, in the professional sector, the assumption is made that patients follow management protocols and take medications as prescribed. Frequently, however, the authors are aware that patients often have culturally constructed reasons for not complying with protocols or medications, yet are not willing to reveal them to the provider unless they are given an opening to discuss it by the provider. Assessment data would include such things as a patient's specific fears about pain medication, expectations about what he or she thinks the medication will do, goals for pain levels, activities to achieve, and evaluating communication with family and coworkers. The deeper the provider's understanding about research evidence and the more extensive his or her clinical expertise, the more anticipatory guidance the provider can give. In a review of literature on patients' beliefs about pain medication, Monsivais and McNeill[23] found that many patients preferred to avoid taking pain medication whenever possible, which often leads to noncompliance with medication treatment. Although patients may not discuss the fact that they do not want to take pain medication, knowledgable providers may in effect have to give patients "permission" to take it, and emphasize that rehabilitation will be enhanced if they follow the medication protocol. Mrs K was willing to take medication in preparation for being active, but did not understand that better pain relief might be achieved if the medication was taken on a routine basis.

Patients who share a chronic condition may be considered a cultural subgroup. Provider expertise with chronic pain patients often means the provider can pick up certain pain-related behaviors that could be considered "cultural cues" related to the chronic pain condition. Somatizing, overdramatization, withholding information, and leaving the system are examples of these pain-related behaviors.[24]

According to the guidelines for the assessment and management of chronic pain,[21] a multidisciplinary team approach that incorporates all facets of the patient's life is needed. This approach would include physical and biologic factors, psychological factors, as well as family, social, and work environment factors. Improved outcomes for chronic pain patients frequently occur when psychosocial problems are properly managed.[25,26] Mrs K would have benefited from a complete assessment by a pain management specialist and the multidisciplinary team approach.

A multifaceted team approach incorporating high levels of evidence, provider expertise, and patient preferences and values sets the stage for "best practice" chronic pain care that will enhance outcomes.

SUMMARY

Understanding how patients construct and make sense of their chronic pain during interactions with the health care system can be considered both as research evidence and as part of provider expertise (see **Fig. 1**). Areas of cultural tensions in chronic pain frequently involve the struggle to achieve credibility regarding one's pain and complying with pain medication protocols.

When individual patient values and preferences are incorporated into the CRCM along with published research findings, providers are able to move toward a model of care that promotes cultural competency for patients with chronic pain.

REFERENCES

1. Morris DB. Illness and culture in the postmodern age. Berkeley (CA): University of California Press; 1998.
2. Engebretson J, Littleton LY. Cultural negotiation: a constructivist-based model for nursing practice. Nurs Outlook 2001;49(5):223–30.
3. Kleinman A. Writing at the margin: discourse between anthropology and medicine. Arthur Kleinman. 260 Berkeley (CA): University of California Press; 1995. 300 Xiii, p. 314, 24 Cm.
4. Eccleston C, Williams AC, Rogers WS. Patients' and professionals' understandings of the causes of chronic pain: Blame, responsibility and identity protection. Soc Sci Med 1997;45(5):699–709.
5. Kenny DT. Constructions of chronic pain in doctor-patient relationships: bridging the communication chasm. Patient Educ Couns 2004;52(3):297–305.
6. Johansson EE, Hamberg K, Lindgren G, et al. "I've been crying my way"—qualitative analysis of a group of female patients' consultation experiences. Fam Pract 1996;13(6):498–503.
7. Johansson EE, Hamberg K, Westman G, et al. The meanings of pain: an exploration of women's descriptions of symptoms. Soc Sci Med 1999;48(12):1791–802.
8. Tait RC, Chibnall JT. Physician judgments of chronic pain patients. Soc Sci Med 1997;45(8):1199–205.
9. Peters S, Stanley I, Rose M, et al. Patients with medically unexplained symptoms: sources of patients' authority and implications for demands on medical care. Soc Sci Med 1998;46(4–5):559–65.

10. Harding G, Parsons S, Rahman A, et al. It struck me that they didn't understand pain: the specialist pain clinic experience of patients with chronic musculoskeletal pain. Arthritis Rheum 2005;53(5):691–6.
11. Monsivais D. Self-organization in chronic pain: a concept analysis. Rehabil Nurs 2005;30(4):147–51.
12. Ponte CD, Johnson-Tribino J. Attitudes and knowledge about pain: an assessment of West Virginia family physicians. Fam Med 2005;37(7):477–80.
13. O'Rorke JE, Chen I, Genao I, et al. Physicians' comfort in caring for patients with chronic nonmalignant pain. Am J Med Sci 2007;333(2):93–100.
14. Weiner DK, Turner GH, Hennon JG, et al. The state of chronic pain education in geriatric medicine fellowship training programs: results of a national survey. J Am Geriatr Soc 2005;53(10):1798–805.
15. Tarzian AJ, Hoffmann DE. Barriers to managing pain in the nursing home: findings from a statewide survey. J Am Med Dir Assoc 2005;6(Suppl 3):S13–9.
16. Parsons S, Harding G, Breen A, et al. The influence of patients' and primary care practitioners' beliefs and expectations about chronic musculoskeletal pain on the process of care: a systematic review of qualitative studies. Clin J Pain 2007;23(1): 91–8.
17. Breuer B, Cruciani R, Portenoy RK. Pain management by primary care physicians, pain physicians, chiropractors, and acupuncturists: a national survey. South Med J 2010;103(8):738–47.
18. Monsivais DB. Understanding cultural constructions of chronic pain in Mexican-American women. ProQuest Digital Dissertations 2008 (AAT3362677).
19. Patton MQ. Qualitative research & evaluation methods. 3rd edition. Thousand Oaks (CA): Sage Publications; 2002.
20. Engebretson J, Mahoney J, Carlson E. Cultural competency in the era of evidence-based practice. J Prof Nurs 2008;24(3):172–8.
21. Cross T, Bazron B, Dennis K, et al. Towards a culturally competent system of care, vol. 1. Child and Adolescent Service System Program Technical Assistance Center. Washington DC: Georgetown University Child Development Center; 1989.
22. Registered Nurses Association of Ontario (RNAO). Assessment and management of pain. Toronto (ON): Registered Nurses Association of Ontario (RNAO); 2002. p. 142 and Registered Nurses Association of Ontario (RNAO). Assessment and management of pain: supplement. Toronto (ON): Registered Nurses Association of Ontario (RNAO); 2007. p. 27. Available at: http://www.guideline.gov/content.aspx?id=11507&search=rnao. Accessed September 22, 2010.
23. Monsivais D, McNeill J. Multicultural influences on pain medication attitudes and beliefs in patients with nonmalignant chronic pain syndromes. Pain Manag Nurs 2007;8(2):64–71.
24. Monsivais D, Engebretson J. Cultural cues: review of qualitative evidence of patient-centered care in patients with non-malignant chronic pain. Rehabil Nurs, in press.
25. Monsivais JJ, Robinson K. Psychological profile and work status of a predominantly Hispanic worker's compensation population with chronic limb pain. Hand (N Y) 2008;3(4):352–8.
26. Rosenberger PH, Jokl P, Ickovics J. Psychosocial factors and surgical outcomes: an evidence-based literature review. J Am Acad Orthop Surg 2006;14(7): 397–405.

Culturally Competent Care for Parkinson Disease

Melinda Hermanns, PhD, RN, BC, CNE

KEYWORDS

- Parkinson disease • Clinically Relevant Continuum Model
- Culturally competent care

Parkinson disease (PD) is a devastating and disabling disease that interferes with a person's ability to perform routine activities of daily living.[1] An estimated 1 million Americans witness the daily effects of this neurodegenerative disorder.[2] PD is a complex, mysterious disorder with a high degree of individual variation. PD may take 20 years or more to develop in some, whereas in others, the progression may be much more rapid. Nevertheless, PD can transform people with little or no disability to total impairment over the progressive stages of the disease. Although the cause is known, it is not well understood, but researchers continue to search for a treatment and possible cure. The goal of treatment is generally palliative, with the administration of antiparkinsonian agents and/or surgery. Deep brain stimulation (DBS) is a surgical procedure that is used when symptoms cannot be adequately managed by medication. DBS has been fairly successful in controlling the physical manifestations of the disease.[3]

Although substantial information is known about the pathophysiology, little is known about the patient's illness experience of living with PD.[4] With 50,000 individuals diagnosed with PD annually,[2] the paucity of research on the experience of living with a neurodegenerative disorder is significant. Most of the research in PD focuses on the biomedical approach to care that supports traditional medical interventions. Few qualitative studies have been located that examine the illness experience.[5] In addition to the biomedical research, other studies have focused on the psychosocial experience of the patient[6] and the caregiver perspective[7] using self-report instruments.

The collective evidence reinforces the idea that the chronic illness experience is embedded in the structural realities and cultural knowledge inherent in the social world of the patient.[4] The current understanding of the illness experience in chronic disease

The author has nothing to disclose.
College of Nursing and Health Sciences, The University of Texas at Tyler, 3900 University Boulevard, Tyler, TX 75799, USA
E-mail address: mhermanns@uttyler.edu

has been shaped by the contributions of an array of academic disciplines. Epidemiologically, the illness experience is viewed as the number of people sharing a specific chronic disease in a given population. Psychologically, the literature has focused on coping and adaptation and other related psychological disturbances. Socially, evidence has examined the role of chronic illness and its affect on human relationships. Philosophically, being sick and staying sick have 2 distinct meanings. Anthropologist Arthur Kleinman[8] cogently differentiated the meaning of disease and illness. The disease is what the physician treats, and the illness is what the patient lives and experiences. PD is complex and multifaceted, making the subjective experience difficult to examine. Kleinman[9] advocated for eliciting the illness experience, which encompasses the explanation models that reveal how patients understand their disease. These applications to persons with PD can help to further understand the pragmatic issues of living with this chronic, progressive disorder.

Anecdotal testimonies substantiate that chronic illnesses have a major effect on one's daily life and illuminate the importance of understanding the perspective of the illness experience of the person with the disease.[10] Kleinman[11(p48)] posits "the meanings of chronic illness are created by the sick person and his or her circle to make over a wild, disordered natural occurrence into a more or less domesticated mythologized, ritually controlled, therefore cultural experience."

The data reported in this article were part of a larger study that sought to understand how people with PD construct their illness experience and manage living with PD on a daily basis.[5] This article focuses on the individual and the group descriptions of their explanatory models (EMs) of people with PD describe their disease in terms of identification and causation, which are based on Kleinman and Benson's[12] EMs that include a description naming, causation, understanding what happens to the person with the disease, prognosis or course of the disease, and what one might do to make it better. The application of the Clinically Relevant Continuum Model is also discussed as a means of promoting culturally competent care in a group of individuals who share a common cultural experience, PD.

METHOD

Denzin and Lincoln[13] proposed that human experiences about which little is known, as in the case of meaningful construction of the illness experience in persons living with the disease on a day-to-day basis, is best suited for qualitative inquiry. In the larger study, an ethnographic approach was used in an attempt to understand how people experience, describe, and interpret their illness experience in their daily life.[5] Data were collected from fieldwork and long semistructured interviews. In the larger study, the illness experience was captured by the personal accounts of 7 men and 7 women with PD. The 3 content themes were PD and the Impact on the Self: The Reflective Process, Daily Negotiations in the Midst of Uncertainty, and the Impact of the Transitioning Self on Day-to-Day Existence. The metaphor, "sailing the sea in the eye of the storm" was used to depict their voyage of living with PD.[5]

The analysis for this report is based on Kleinman's[9] work on EMs. Kleinman's original approach to medical anthropology involved an exploratory process of qualitative inquiry and examined how clinical reality exists in the minds of health care professionals and patients. This ethnographic interview approach leads to complex and multilayered responses that carry with them information about social rituals, symbols in communication, forms of knowledge, and illness narratives. Kleinman perceived the clinical reality of the patient as consisting of psychological reality, biological reality, and physical reality. He termed the patient's reality and cultural or societal reality the "symbolic reality." Health care professionals who endeavor to understand a patient's symbolic reality can potentially tap into individuals' rich view of the world and their experience of illness within that world. Kleinman labels these reflective processes as effects to an individual as EMs of illness. Using this holistic and reflective language may give patients a window of understanding their suffering even without the potential for recovery. EMs can be investigated through the use of socioanthropological research strategies of participant observation and individual and group open-ended conversations. Kleinman and Benson[12] identified a specific area of conical ethnography as contrasting the patient's EMs of disease with the biomedical model. Western health care professionals tend to be oriented to descriptions of disease, thus focusing on the diagnosis and treatment rather than the patient's total experience of the illness.[8] Patients' constructions, on the other hand, are oriented to illness as an individual and shared process. Spradley[14] contends that people with a shared experience become a culturally defined social group.

SAMPLE

Fieldwork was conducted in East Texas over a 2-year period. The sites for fieldwork were 2 PD support groups in East Texas. This study purposively sampled persons in the various stages of PD in an attempt to illuminate the illness experience. In addition, purposively sampling was used to allow access to patient groups in settings that were related to the health care system and also support groups that were patients and family. The sample of key informants selected for the long individual interviews included 14 participants with PD and attendees of 2 local PD support groups. According to Spradley,[14] human experiences from a cultural perspective are an important aspect to understand the lives of others within contextual realities and from their own native point of view.

ETHICAL CONSIDERATIONS

Ethics approval was obtained from university committees as well as letters of support from the neurology offices, PD support groups, and hospital affiliates. Written consent was obtained after informing participants of the study the purpose and their role in the research.

DATA COLLECTION AND ANALYSIS

Detailed field notes were kept by the researcher on each interview and field observation session. Field notes were dictated immediately following the interviews and support group experiences in an effort to capture pertinent thoughts and reflections.

INTERVIEWS

The narrative interview is the most common method of qualitative data collection and is well suited to explicating how individuals make meaning of their life and illness experience.[13] Structured interviews focused on how persons with PD construct their illness experience and manage living with the disease. Interviews lasted approximately 30 minutes to 1.5 hours. Open-ended questions and probes were incorporated in an attempt to elicit rich descriptions of participants' experiences.[15]

All interviews were tape-recorded and transcribed verbatim and, along with field notes, thematic analysis was conducted. Once data were collected, the researcher reviewed each transcript, identifying salient thematic content in each profile and substantiating the common meaning structures with participants' verbatim accounts, and compared with field notes as a means of developing coding and categories. Two years of fieldwork was conducted, and comments from the 14 individual interviews as well as the attendees of the PD support groups relative to the individual and groups' naming and causation of the disease are reported.

FINDINGS

Findings fell into 2 overlapping categories, those similar to the components of Kleinman and Benson's[12] EM. These were Constructing the Disease and Causation and Their Quest for Knowledge. This interpretation of experience has been termed the worldview of an individual or group.[15]

CONSTRUCTING THE DISEASE

The EM developed by people with PD was a beginning point for the researcher to understand their view of reality. Participant constructions provided the researcher with a clinical biomedical description of the disease itself, but a deeper meaning was needed to better understand the subjective construction of their illness experience.

Once the researcher established initial rapport, the participants were extremely forthcoming in discussing their disease. All of the participants openly shared the process by which they labeled their disease. Mr H was selected as an exemplar case. Mr H talked about his journey of constructing/naming his disease. Before the formal medical diagnosis of PD, he began to experience subtle symptoms of tremor in his hands and dragging of his feet, all of which became increasingly noticeable and hugely annoying. On his awareness of his initial symptoms, he and his wife started reading about various neurologic disorders that may have accounted for his symptoms as he admitted to the enjoyment of reading and his passion for learning. In his living room, the researcher noticed an extensive collection of encyclopedias and a computer with Internet access, which they both stated that they used. It was not long before they became convinced that he had PD. He made an appointment with his local medical doctor who referred him to a neurologist, at which time their suspicion of PD was confirmed. Although he had associated his symptoms with the diagnosis of PD, hearing the diagnosis was devastating; there were no longer any doubts; he indeed had PD. Mr H did not have a family history of PD nor did he know anyone with the disease. In talking with Mr H, the biomedical discourse of PD as a neurologic disease with its unique pathophysiology, epidemiology, and symptoms was identified as the major focus in his responses.

Mr H's responses were in line with Kleinman's EM in that he integrated the professional sector, that is, the health care professional's understanding, into his own explanation. In this study, he was given an opportunity to talk about PD from his perspective in an effort to understand his construction of his illness experience. He acknowledged that this was difficult because no one had ever asked him to explain PD in his own terms. Mr H's experience was similar to Murphy's[16] narrative of his illness experience of being disabled. Murphy explicitly stated that no one ever asked him what it was like to be paraplegic; rather, the focus of the health care professionals was objective, clinical and focused on the mechanisms of the disease not the perspective of the person with the illness. Mr H cogently described PD as a disease that is always there, with the symptoms serving as a constant reminder that he has the disease. He was aware that PD is a progressive disorder and that it will get worse over time. He was knowledgeable about his symptoms and medications, sharing ways in which he adjusted his medications according to his symptoms.

In terms of naming the disease, participants used a variety of terminologies. Echoed in the support group was the language they used to describe PD: a brain disease, a neurologic disorder. The predominant use of medical terminology served as their means of communicating with each other about their disease and symptoms, for example, tremor, freezing, rigidity, and may indicate the group's cultural orientation to the biomedical facilities. Many talked about their symptoms, and no 2 persons with PD were the same. Participant beliefs of having a uniquely personal experience of the illness are illustrated by these comments:

You can't compare your symptoms to another person.
No two people with Parkinson's are the same.

In addition, the symptoms and the individual illness experience may further contribute to the complexity of PD and highlight the importance of examining how persons with chronic diseases cognitively construct their world.

CAUSATION: THEIR QUEST FOR KNOWLEDGE

The 14 participants and the support group attendees shared similar attempts in their quest to learn about what caused their PD. Many admitted that they were not otherwise familiar with PD before their formal diagnosis. Once diagnosed, they shared that they used a variety of sources in their quest for knowledge. Most admitted that they reverted to books, magazines, and the Internet in an attempt to identify a cause. Yet, most stated that they considered their physician and nurse practitioner as a reliable source of information and asked the trusted professionals to explain the causation. All were on a quest to find knowledge, some explanation, an answer to "what caused my PD?" Evidence substantiates that communication between provider and client is essential.[17] When there are differences in the understanding of the illness, communication suffers and adherence to treatment decreases.

PD was frequently referred to as a mysterious disorder because the cause of PD was unknown. Individual and group discussions about possible causes included thoughts of living in rural areas in which well water was the primary source of water, the use of pesticides on crops, and childhood trauma involving an automobile accident. Many of the participants did not have a family history of PD; in contrast, Mrs C's mother and aunt died of PD. Mrs C was identified as an exemplar case. Despite her familiarity with the symptoms of PD from family observations as well as observations in a long, varied career in the medical field, she was dismayed and skeptical when the original diagnosis of PD was made. Mrs C's constructions of PD stemmed from witnessing her mother and aunt's physical and mental decline. Conversely, Mr H did not have a history of PD. Mr H shared an enlightening preliminary encounter years before he was diagnosed with PD. His inspiring story is as follows: Mr H was asked by one of the ministers at his church if he would mind picking up a lady who could not longer drive to church because of her PD. Mr H was willing to help, as he would take her to church every week for more than a year until at which time, her PD had progressed to the point that she was no longer able to ride in the car. She became homebound and required nursing assistance. At that point, he continued to visit her, dropping off sermon tapes of the church service. Mr H talked about how it was difficult to see this dear lady's condition deteriorate, but was happy that he was able to help her. Years later, Mr H was diagnosed with PD. He recalled all the times he had driven that special lady with PD to church. Mr H said that he thought it was God's way of preparing him of what was to come, his diagnosis of PD. Although Mr H did not have a family history of PD, he thought that his cause was ordained by God.

In addition to naming the disease and attempting to identify the cause, participants were asked to describe a typical day. The concept of daily negotiation in the larger study came to light when a participant could not describe a typical day.

Parkinson's dictates my day. I mean there are days that I feel good and I want to get out and just go, go, go, but my body just won't work. My mind tells my body to go but it doesn't listen. It does me no good to plan things, because I never know what I am physically going to be able to do on any given day.

Similar responses included comments such as "I don't have any consistent days" and "My world revolves around a clock and the effectiveness of my medicine." In addition, many of the participants admitted that the physical symptoms of PD, specifically tremors, lack of coordination and balance, and freezing, kept them from a variety of activities at certain times. Their day-to-day activities revolved around how they felt and their medication regimen. Daily living requires minute-to-minute decision-making skills. Questions such as "Can I button my shirt?" and "Am I going to able to cook breakfast for myself?" are all daily realities. These statements reflect Kleinman's EMs that ask "what is happening to my body" and "what is the course of the disease." The realization that there was *no* typical day prevailed in all 14 participants. Day-to-day, often minute-to-minute, assessments depending on their PD symptoms and the effectiveness of their medication dictated their day. Mrs D responded:

It is frustrating. You can't do what you normally want to do or like I can't tie my shoe sometimes. Now I am to the point that I can't get dressed without help. Everything that I go to do is hard to do. Getting the lids off of jars or opening a box or trying to read or anything I do is more difficult...Things you just take for granted until you can't do it.

Sitting at the support group meetings, it became increasingly clear that their activities revolved around their medication schedule. The participants have to deal with their changing self in living with a progressive disorder and the simultaneous negotiation of day-to-day activities for daily living. They all admitted that they had to learn how to manage their disease. All of the participants talked about what they could do to make their PD better, stating that "resting makes it better," and when asked what makes it worse, the overwhelming response was "getting in a hurry." This response was also echoed in the informal discussions at the support groups. They all shared that they absolutely could not get in a hurry or get stressed out; "I don't sweat the small stuff." Often, they have to "sit and wait" for the medication to take effect. Although a sense of relief was felt among all when a diagnosis was determined, the unknown cause of PD remained a mystery. Many still question the cause of their PD and thus continue to seek information about PD.

Ultimately, the participants were forced to admit their physical weaknesses and seek a new identity in an effort to experience a reconstructed self with PD.[5] The idea of a threatened identity seems to be in line with Charmaz's[18(p674)] research on chronic illness, in which the author states, "chronic illness attacks the body and threatens the integrity of self." Charmaz[18(p675)] stated, "...ill people paradoxically grow more resolute in self as they adapt to impairment; they suffer bodily losses but gain themselves." Although PD was a threat to all of the participants interviewed, their strong faith, attitude, and sense of wholeness was identified as their stronghold in preserving the self. In summary, PD challenges one's life, life as they knew it and in essence, all that their lives have stood for, but many found a way to fit PD into an overall schema of a meaningful life.[5]

The way in which one reflects on the self can have a vital effect on the cognitive constructions of the illness experience as seen in the 14 participants in the larger study.[5] Their ability to reflect on their illness experience as well as the process of reassessing who they are and who they can become seemed to aid in their ability to accommodate to the physical losses and reunified body and self fittingly.

DISCUSSION

The professional sector consists of health care professionals and is oriented around the biomedical model, in which the focus is on the medical treatment. The Clinically Relevant Continuum Model[19] recognizes the patient values and circumstances, the patient's perspective of their illness, and treatment, which results in a more holistic and comprehensive approach to care as well as effective communication and interventions. Addressing patient values and circumstances is the key to cultural competency. Culturally competent care requires a commitment from the health care professions as well as other caregivers to understand and be attentive to the cultural needs of others, that is, be culturally sensitive. It is important for nurses to be culturally competent; understanding and effectively communicating with the patients ensure the best possible clinical outcome.

The ability to provide culturally competent care is especially important for practicing nurses who function in a variety of roles in the health care environment. Nurses must develop cultural competency to be effective in establishing rapport with patients and to accurately assess, develop, and implement nursing interventions designed to meet patients' needs. When a cultural perspective contradicts mainstream health care practices, we must advocate for our patients and support the patient's and family's decisions. Therefore, nurses must have a clear understanding of the various cultures to be able to deliver culturally competent care to all patients. The process of seeking to understand cultural perspectives is the key to gaining knowledge, understanding, and appreciation of cultural values.[20]

Although most research in PD has focused on the biomedical disease and treatment, extensive quantitative clinical research on the disease process, together with this ethnographic study and other qualitative studies, may assist health care professions in evidence-based practice. Cultural competency involves being attuned to cultural cues the patient and family present during the clinical encounter regarding attitudes and beliefs about illness, behaviors, treatment expectations, and family response to the person who is ill. Culture refers to the values and beliefs underlying behaviors held by a group of people. Thus, groups who negotiate living in a society with a particular chronic condition can be considered cultural subgroups sharing elements of a common experience, such as in this ethnographic study, the subgroup consisted of individuals who live in East Texas, sharing a diagnosis of PD. Their experience illuminated the cultural issues in PD and represents a subset of the population specific to East Texas.

Researchers have come to regard persons with chronic illness as experts in their own feelings, concerns, and experiences.[21] Phillips[22] contends the way in which persons incorporate PD into the ability to maintain personal control in their life, thereby emphasizing the desire to maintain control over one's life as long as possible. The patients' rich view of the world and of their illness within the world gives rise to a better understanding of their illness experience, including its meaning to the self and the healing process.[16] Nurses may assist patients in the development of their own EM to elicit the patient's perspective of illness, thus challenging the explanatory paradigm of medicine, which has a predominantly biomedical model. Exploration of the patient and nurses' EMs is valuable in developing culturally capable nursing practice. The participants' construction of their illness experience through the development of their own EM and their process of encountering, processing, and integrating information yielded a greater understanding of their illness, including its meaning to them and their illness experience. Understanding the illness experience as constructed by the patient may facilitate the communication between the popular and professional sectors. This understanding and enhanced communication may influence the future care provided to persons with PD.

Findings from the works of Brod and colleagues[23] and Abudi and colleagues[24] support the idea that persons' perception and experience of their PD vary from the professional's perception, thus emphasizing the need for further exploration of the patients' view of their illness experience. "The ways that an individual or group of people label an illness and seek and evaluate treatment are embedded in a cultural system that provides not only for the interpretation of an illness but also for the rules and rituals of illness behavior."[18(p658)] One of the beauties of using the Clinically Relevant Continuum Model[19] is that it supports a partnership between the health care provider and the individual in an effort to provide comprehensive and best possible care. The existing paradigm of nursing care in PD may be challenged through the delivery of a whole-person approach to care, for example, a holistic approach, and giving voice to the individual affected by the disease. Engebretson and Littleton[25(p223)] state, "The holistic approach involves understanding the interrelationships of the biologic, psychologic, sociocultural, and spiritual dimensions of the person who is interacting with internal and external components of the environment." More qualitative studies are needed to develop new knowledge in understanding how individuals make meaning of their disease and integrate their illness experience into daily life.

IMPLICATIONS

The implications for further research suggested by the findings of this study are several. Future research needs to focus on the whole-body approach (biological, psychological, social, and spiritual aspects) and the individual's adaptation to a chronic, progressive disease. Explicit descriptions of the theoretical underpinnings as well as the use of a conceptual framework and models such as the Clinically Relevant Continuum Model are strongly recommended in an effort to guide research in understanding PD.

SUMMARY

Delivering culturally competent care implies a contextual understanding that treating the illness and understanding what it means to the individual are as important to resolve as the disease process. The transition from illness experience to disorder is determined by social decision points rather than a biomedical focus of the disorder. An approach to learning local systems of EMs, which are common to specific cultural groups, needs to be achieved. In light of culturally complex clinical presentations, exploration of the patient and clinician's EM is valuable in developing a culturally capable nursing practice. Using the Clinically Relevant Continuum Model promotes a more holistic approach in the delivery of patient-centered care.[19] If the provision of the best possible care for all patients is the goal, practicing nurses must have expertise and skill in the delivery of culturally appropriate and culturally competent nursing care. The delivery of culturally competent care that fosters effective interactions and the development of appropriate responses may be a challenge but is vital to effectively care for persons with PD.

REFERENCES

1. Lee AJ. Problems in diagnosis. In: Factor SA, Weiner WJ, editors. Parkinson's disease: diagnosis and clinical management. New York: Demos; 2002. p. 243–50.
2. Parkinson's Disease Foundation. About Parkinson's page. Available at: http://www.pdf.org/AboutPD/. Updated January 31, 2010. Accessed October 31, 2010.
3. Piper M, Abrams GM, Marks WJ Jr. Deep brain stimulation for the treatment of Parkinson's disease: overview and impact on gait and mobility. NeuroRehabilitation 2005;20(3):223–32.
4. Thorne S, Paterson B, Acorn B, et al. Chronic illness experience: insights from a metastudy. Qual Health Res 2002;12:437–52.
5. Stanley-Hermanns M. The illness experience of persons with Parkinson's disease. (The University of Texas Health Science Center at Houston doctoral dissertation). ETD collection for Houston Academy of Medicine-Texas Medical Center; 2008. Paper AAI3308879.
6. Backer J. The symptom experience of patients with Parkinson's disease: review of literature. J Neurosci Nurs 2006;38(1):51–7.
7. Maier K, Calne S. Informal caregivers: a valuable part of the health care team. In: Manuchair E, Pfeiffer R, editors. Parkinson's disease. London: Taylor & Francis; 2006. p. 999–1008.
8. Kleinman A. Patients and healers in the context of culture. Berkeley (CA): University of California Press; 1980. p. 85–6.
9. Kleinman A. Interpreting illness experience and clinical meanings: how I see clinically applied anthropology. Med Anthropol Q 1985;16(3):69–71.
10. Frank A. The wounded storyteller. Chicago: The University of Chicago Press; 1995. p. 1–27.
11. Kleinman A. The illness narratives: suffering, healing and the human condition. New York: Basic Books, Incorporated; 1988. p. 3–30; 48.
12. Kleinman A, Benson P. Anthropology in the clinic: the problem of cultural competency and how to fix it. PLoS Med 2006;3(10):1673–6.
13. Denzin NK, Lincoln Y. The discipline and practice of qualitative research. In: Denzin N, Lincoln Y, editors. Handbook of qualitative research. Thousand Oaks (CA): Sage; 2008. p. 1–29.
14. Spradley JP. In: Doing participant observation. Participant observation. New York: Holt, Rinehart, and Winston; 1980. p. 53–8.
15. Creswell JW. Five qualitative traditions of inquiry. In: Creswell JW, editor. Qualitative inquiry and research design: choosing among five traditions. Thousand Oaks (CA): Sage Publications, Incorporated; 1998. p. 34–5.
16. Murphy RF. The Struggle for Autonomy. In: The body silent. New York: WW Norton; 1990. p. 5–16 [Chapter: 6].
17. Neuman B. Resonating the whole. In: Transforming presence: the difference that nursing makes. Philadelphia: FA Davis; 2008. p. 33–50 [Chapter: 4].
18. Charmaz K. The body, identity, and self: adapting to impairment. Sociol Q 1995; 36(4):657–80.
19. Engebretson J, Mahoney J, Carlson B. Cultural competence in the era of evidence-based practice. J Prof Nurs 2008;24(3):172–8.

20. Campinha-Bacote J. The quest for cultural competence in nursing care. Nurs Forum 1995;30(4):19.

21. Kennedy I. Patients are experts in their own field. BMJ 2003;326:1276–7.

22. Phillips L. Dropping the bomb: the experience of being diagnosed with Parkinson's disease. Geriatr Nurs 2006;27(6):362–9.

23. Brod M, Mendelsohn GA, Roberts B. Patients' experiences of Parkinson's disease. J Gerontol B Psychol Sci Soc Sci 1998;53B(4):213–22.

24. Abudi S, Bar-Tal Y, Ziv L, et al. Parkinson's disease symptoms-patients' perceptions. J Adv Nurs 1997;2(5):54–9.

25. Engebretson J, Littleton LY. Cultural negotiation: a constructivist-based model for nursing practice. Nurs Outlook 2001;40:223–30.

How do Rural Health Care Providers and Patients View Barriers to Colorectal Cancer Screening? Insights from Appalachian Kentucky

Jennifer Hatcher, RN, PhD[a],*, Mark B. Dignan, PhD, MPH[b],
Nancy Schoenberg, PhD[c]

KEYWORDS

- Appalachian Kentucky • Colorectal cancer • Colonoscopy
- Rural

Kentucky has the second highest cancer death rate in the United States, with colorectal cancer (CRC) being one of the leading contributors to that excess mortality rate.[1] The cancer burden for the rural Appalachian population, which comprises 54 of the 120 counties in Kentucky, is even higher than that of Kentucky in general. For the period 2000 to 2005, the age-adjusted mortality rate from all cancers for Kentucky is 222.1/100,000, compared with 235.1/100,000 for the Appalachian region of the state.[2] CRC is also notable because mortality rates are elevated in Kentucky for both sexes. Furthermore, CRC screening represents an ideal opportunity to focus cancer control on both primary and secondary prevention as screening allows for detection and removal of colorectal polyps before they progress to cancer as well as early cancers themselves. Although screening guidelines for CRC are widely

This work was supported by a grant from the National Cancer Institute # CA 11932.
The authors have nothing to disclose.
[a] College of Nursing, University of Kentucky; Lexington, Kentucky; 760 Rose Street, Lexington, KY 40536, USA
[b] Department of Internal Medicine, University of Kentucky College of Medicine, CC444 Roach Facility Markey Center, Lexington, KY 40536, USA
[c] Department of Behavioral Science, University of Kentucky College of Medicine, 125 College of Medicine Office Building, Lexington, KY 40536, USA
* Corresponding author.
E-mail address: Jennifer.hatcher@uky.edu

publicized, US screening rates remain extremely low with the Centers for Disease Control reporting that fewer than 40% of CRC cases are found early.[3]

CRC screening rates are low in Appalachia for a number of reasons. Appalachia, particularly the central Appalachian region that includes Kentucky, suffers from higher unemployment, fewer college graduates, higher poverty rates, lower levels of health insurance coverage, greater shortages of health care providers, and underfinanced health services. These factors have been found to have a significant negative impact on screening rates.[4] In addition, access to health care services, particularly the specialty care needed to provide endoscopic CRC screening tests, is limited in the Appalachian region. Behavioral Risk Factor Surveillance System survey data indicate that Kentuckians aged 50 years and older are less likely to report having had a blood stool test within the past 2 years (24% compared with 26.5% nationwide) than residents of other states.[3] For flexible sigmoidoscopy or colonoscopy, the difference in self-reported screening is more pronounced, with 47.2% of Kentucky respondents reporting ever having either flexible sigmoidoscopy or colonoscopy compared with 53.5% for the United States respondents. Because low screening rates are associated with elevated mortality rates, improved understanding of factors that impede screening is a key element in reducing mortality.

Few studies have examined the unique barriers to CRC screening for rural Appalachians. Wackerbarth and colleagues[5] explored the factors that influence decision making regarding CRC screening among persons in non-Appalachian Kentucky. They conducted 30 semistructured interviews with screened and unscreened persons between the ages of 48 and 55 years. Ten themes emerged from their research representing a wide range of concerns, including structural issues, the nature of the screening tests, individual's health beliefs, and psychological issues. The researchers suggested as a next step that these findings be compared with perspectives of Appalachian residents.

There are also few studies that provide insight into the unique perspective of health care providers regarding CRC screening in this part of the country.[6] Researchers used mixed methods to explore the perceptions of providers and staff from 5 primary care practices in rural Appalachian Kentucky. These health care providers participated in focus groups and completed surveys regarding the CRC screening practices of the patients in their practices. Physician/practice barriers included limited time, more pressing medical concerns, and reimbursement issues. They perceived the patient issues to include fear and embarrassment as primary barriers. In addition, providers questioned the importance of following US Preventive Services Task Force guidelines versus using personal experience when recommending screening for this population, given many of their unique circumstances and beliefs. This article explores the attitudes and beliefs concerning CRC screening among patients and health care providers in rural Appalachian Kentucky. The findings will be useful in developing culturally acceptable interventions to promote CRC screening among persons in this region.

METHODS
Setting

This study was conducted in rural Appalachian Kentucky (**Fig. 1**). This region has long been characterized by picturesque mountainous terrain, but limited road systems, isolation, high rates of poverty, and poor health.[7] Even though conditions have improved since the "War on Poverty" and other "Great Society" programs that were initiated in the 1960s, economic, educational, and health disparities persist.[8] The

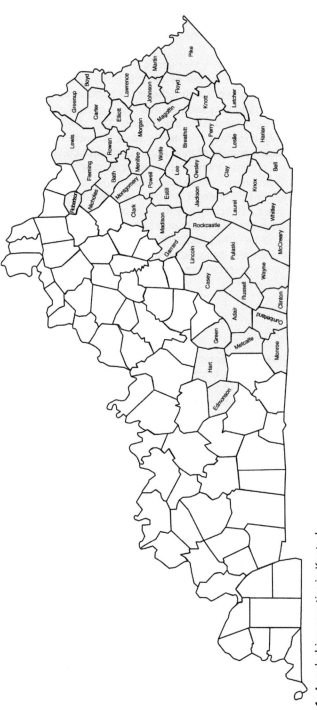

Fig. 1. Appalachian counties in Kentucky.

condition of the health care delivery system in Appalachian Kentucky is consistent with the economic conditions in the region. There has been a chronic shortage of health care providers, and the services that are provided are often underfinanced. As a result, provision of preventive health services falls heavily on the public health system.[9,10]

To elicit a broad range of factors that shape perceptions about screening for CRC from the provider and patient points of view, 5 focus groups were conducted: 3 with primary care providers and 2 with patients. In addition to exploring the barriers to CRC screening according to guidelines, the focus groups elicited preferences for particular screening modalities among participants. The providers were asked about methods of enhancing screening in practice environments. The authors elected to undertake focus groups because of their potential to capture unrehearsed thoughts, feelings, and opinions and capitalize on the discussions of others.[11,12]

Primary care providers were included because of their critical role in the screening process, and because health care in Appalachian Kentucky is provided mostly by primary care providers. Specialists who perform colorectal screening (flexible sigmoidoscopy or colonoscopy) are in short supply. Provider recommendation has been demonstrated to be a key factor in encouraging patients to obtain cancer screening.[13] To enhance the generalizability of the findings, the authors chose to conduct focus groups with providers and patients in several different geographic areas of Appalachian Kentucky.

SAMPLE AND RECRUITMENT

The authors used theoretical sampling, selecting participants on the basis of their potential ability to contribute to issues at hand, rather than attempting to recruit a representative sample.[14] To garner a full range of input, they included different types of relevant health care providers (nurses, general practice physicians, specialists, office managers) in a variety of practice settings (private clinics, local health departments, federally qualified community health centers) and involved a broad cross section of participants (varying in income, education, occupation, health status).

Participants were recruited for the 3 provider focus groups through letters and follow-up telephone calls. The process began with development of a list of providers compiled through interactions with the Kentucky Medical Association and Kentucky Medical Licensure databases. The research team reviewed the list, and a diverse group of providers was contacted to participate in the study. The sample was selected to ensure geographic representation, to include providers in both solo and group practice, and to limit selection to those in adult primary care (general practice, family medicine, and general internal medicine).

Patient focus group participants were recruited through posting announcements in clinic waiting rooms and with the assistance of a community advisory board. Community advisory board members disseminated information about the focus groups through social and civic groups and worksites. Two patient focus groups were conducted, one with those who had undergone screening within the past year and one with those who had been rarely (not within the past 5 years) or never screened for CRC. The groups were organized by screening status to make sure that the views of unscreened individuals were captured, as prior research suggests that the views of screened and unscreened persons may differ in important ways.[15] On acceptance of the authors' invitation to join a luncheon or dinner and discussion of CRC issues, a convenient location and time were arranged.

Data Collection

On arrival, investigators greeted focus group participants, administered informed consent procedures, and answered all questions or concerns. After these activities, the authors administered a brief sociodemographic questionnaire. The moderator then provided a general introduction to the focus group process, followed by a series of open-ended questions focusing on the barriers to CRC screening, knowledge of and perspectives about the various screening techniques, and, for the providers, methods of increasing screening in practices. The discussions lasted approximately 60 to 120 minutes, depending on the level of detail provided by the participants and the group dynamics. All protocols and procedures were approved by the institutional review board at the University of Kentucky.

Data Processing and Analysis

All sessions were tape recorded and professionally transcribed. Two qualitatively trained researchers independently reviewed the transcripts multiple times, and data were content analyzed. Core categories of emerging substantive findings were identified after conducting line-by-line analysis. These categories guided the initial coding and eventually lead to the development of a codebook.[16] Several iterations of the codebook and repeated discussions on the interpretations of data enhanced the rigor of the process. Qualitative analysis tends to be recursive; thus, data collection, immersion in the transcripts, and subsequent coding and development of a codebook were performed simultaneously.[17]

The authors did not use any qualitative data analysis software; however, they took several additional steps to insure the rigor and trustworthiness of the data analysis. First, the moderators and assistants supplied memo writing and field observations. Second, they conducted member checks with the interview staff, most of whom reside in the Appalachian communities in which the focus groups occurred. Finally, they used coding techniques to enhance the rigor in their data interpretation. Specifically, all of the transcripts were co-coded by at least 2 qualitative researchers using the codebook the authors developed, eventually leading to overall agreement in coding.

RESULTS

The provider focus group participants included primary care physicians, physician assistants, and nurse practitioners. The 2 patient focus groups included participants aged 50 years and older, without a history of CRC and with a variety of education and income levels. A total of 5 focus groups were conducted: 3 with primary care providers and 2 with patients. The primary care provider focus groups ranged in number from 5 to 7 participants. The patient focus groups included 1 group of 6 participants and 1 group of 11. The focus groups were conducted as planned, but although the questions were framed to address general perspectives on CRC screening, each group quickly gravitated toward discussing colonoscopy as the only "good" method of screening for CRC. Thus, in this article, data on provider and nonprovider perspectives on colonoscopy are presented, specifically focusing on perceived merits and limitations of this screening modality.

Results from Primary Care Provider Focus Groups

The providers identified 2 main categories of challenges to rural Appalachian patients' receipt of CRC screening, especially colonoscopy. These include the overall categories of (1) patient characteristics and circumstances and (2) health care delivery factors, including reimbursement issues.

Providers frequently described patient characteristics and circumstances that undermine screening. These characteristics include having multiple diseases that are given higher priority than prevention, patient perceptions of mistrust of the medical establishment, and lack of resources. In a population that tends to suffer from serious, complicated chronic conditions, such as diabetes, chronic obstructive pulmonary disease, and heart disease, prevention is often considered to be of less importance than treatment. The following statements represent provider perspectives on barriers associated with patient characteristics:

"Because they're here for other medical problems and if they are quite sick with their heart or diabetes, you sometimes get so pulled up in that that you forget the preventative things."

"It (screening) has to be physician initiated so you have a large population who has minimal physician contact, then you have those who come in with other concerns at that time, then they don't raise that issue and as physicians, we kind of focus initially on what the chief complaint is at that time."

In addition, the providers felt that there were cultural/attitudinal issues preventing screening, including perceptions that cancer is a death sentence, mistrust of providers other than patients' "own doctor," and lack of "appropriate" priorities. For example, 1 provider noted:

"There's a kind of a cultural thing here. I don't know exactly how to describe it or articulate it. A lot of the people up in here prefer to deal with people they know. I think folks up in this part of the hills are particularly reluctant to go anywhere else unless they absolutely have to."

Providers also recognized that patients' financial concerns, specifically the inability of patients to afford copayments and deductibles, were barriers to CRC screening.

"Without a diagnosis, the insurance won't pay for just a routine colonoscopy or sigmoidoscopy at the very minimum, so that's probably the biggest roadblock ..."

Many providers noted that colonoscopy is so expensive that they do not often recommend it for their patients who lack health insurance, a considerable portion of this patient population. Even for those with health insurance, providers sometimes are reluctant to suggest the procedure, knowing that out of pocket costs may be prohibitive.

"Someone just close to me had one done ... we have insurance and it was still around $300.00 or $400.00 with the deductibles and the copays..."

Providers also pointed to characteristics of the colonoscopy that they felt undermined patient acceptability of screening. In addition to the costs of the procedures, providers believed that many of their patients would find the preparation for the procedure unacceptable or that the procedure itself would deter patients from pursuing colonoscopy.

Another theme that emerged and undermined screening involved health care delivery system barriers, including the lack of reimbursement for CRC screening counseling and the inadequate supply of specialist providers.

"The single most basic thing is that there are little, very few financial rewards for doing it. The, our health care system, just what I said before, isn't set up to encourage preventive care."

"There's no reimbursement for sitting down and discussing all that with the patient."

Yet another theme that emerged involved the inadequate supply of specialist providers capable of undertaking colonoscopy. Lacking gastroenterologists or others who have the specialized training and equipment to perform colonoscopy, patients must seek care outside of their counties. Providers complained that patients had to travel long distances to visit a gastroenterologist.

"Its 45 to 60 minutes to the closest doctor that does them. This requires a great deal of advanced planning, reliable transportation, and acceptance of the hassle and costs associated with traversing mountain roads."

Compounding that, the specialized care often carried a higher co-payment than other services causing financial strain:

"It's difficult for them to travel, difficult for them to pay the co-payment and all that..." Furthermore, providers suggested that so many people lack even a general practice provider that it is unlikely many patients would obtain a referral to a specialist.

Results from Patient Focus Groups

The patient focus groups provided a more expansive description of challenges to colonoscopy than the primary care provider groups. These could broadly be categorized as residing in their own characteristics, features of the screening tests themselves, and provider and health care system factors. Participants conceptualized their own barriers as fear; inadequate knowledge; distrust of the medical system and providers; and to a lesser degree than anticipated, financial limitations; and more pressing health concerns.

Fear and lack of knowledge regarding screening guidelines were viewed as important challenges to patients receiving CRC screening. Many focus group members indicated that they preferred not to know if they had the disease for fear it was a "death sentence." *"Now I also think people are afraid. If they have problems, they're afraid to have it because they're afraid they will have cancer."*

Lack of knowledge and confusion regarding the guidelines surrounding CRC screening were also important factors influencing receipt of screening. People also were uncertain if they needed the test if they did not have a family history of CRC.

"...We don't have a history of that in my family...well it's every other generation. I do emphasize it for them (children), even though I don't think about it for me because there's no history there in my family. If there was a history, I probably would've already had one."

Although patients did mention financial issues, they did not see this as a barrier as much as the other issues surrounding CRC screening; however, patients often felt that the providers were not recommending or offering screening because of lack of financial incentive. One person stated *"they probably don't have the machinery that they can get paid a high price for to get it done."* In addition, if their insurance would not pay, they felt the test was not being recommended. *"They're very picky about that. Can you afford it, because your insurance won't cover it?"*

Finally, as mentioned by providers, patients did not see the test as a priority, given other more pressing health concerns or a general lack of prioritizing physician visits.

"Sometimes with me, it may be because I'm there with another problem and sort of in dire straits and I probably don't catch them at a good time to suggest it...I more or less go to the doctor when I am sick."
"That's probably why I don't get screening. I was raised; don't go to the doctor unless you're sick."

Consistent with the provider focus groups, patients described how perceptions of the test itself undermined screening (discomfort of preparation, embarrassment, lack of conclusiveness). The most commonly cited barrier for patients was the procedure, including the preparation for the test and the embarrassment of having colonoscopy performed. As these patients indicate,

"I just dread the, getting ready for the test and then having the test..."
"You hear so many horror stories and from seeing the procedure done several, many times over myself, I know it can't be pleasant."

Because of the discomfort associated with the test itself, some persons were hoping that a less invasive test would soon be available. *"I've been waiting for that new thing comes along. Where you could swallow it and it takes pictures of you..."*

Limitations inherent in the health care delivery system compounded perceptions that the test is invasive and embarrassing because of the perceived lack of privacy in the rural Appalachian setting. Many patients suggested that this lack of privacy and the limited pool of health care providers increased the likelihood that someone you know might perform this awkward procedure. One person stated that she did not do the test, although she could afford it and knew she should have it done, because *"I have to see those people."* Another stated *"It's not that I'm really embarrassed to have it done. It's just that I don't want them seeing me."* One woman stated, *"...you're laying on the table, not a stitch on anywhere. If I'd have had a bag to put over my head, I'd have put it on."*

There was also concern about the confidentiality of medical information in the community. One person described an experience with having a screening test done and waiting for the results.

"I worried all evening. I mean I can remember walking in and out of the hall, worrying about it and wondering what my results were going to be and I come to work the next morning and one of my coworkers told me all about my results."

In addition, lack of provider recommendation played a crucial role in perceived need for screening. In one focus group of 11 persons, only 1 had a doctor who recommended screening. Many said that the doctor only recommended CRC screening if the patient had a family history or were symptomatic. In addition, CRC screening was not as commonly recommended as other tests:

"I do get letters from my doctor saying, you need the mammogram or your pap smear and you need your cholesterol checked but I have never gotten anything about colorectal cancer."
"I'll mention it to her (physician) and she'll say, well if it's not in your family and you've not had any problems...she's not really said you need to go do that."
"I just had my yearly checkup and she didn't mention it. "
"If you had a family member that had colon cancer, they'd probably push it more."

In sum, the patient/nonprovider focus groups included 3 categories of challenges: patient characteristics, the screening test itself, and the provider or health care system. These concerns seemed to be additive; colonoscopy constitutes a little known and rarely recommended procedure that may prevent a relatively unknown cancer through an unpleasant, unavailable, costly, and inconvenient procedure. Nonproviders expressed concern with issues surrounding the test itself, including privacy issues related to living in a close-knit community with few qualified specialists. Participants also emphasized a lack of screening advocacy on the part of providers, a concern amplified due to more pressing health concerns or even more frequently recommended screening tests such as mammography.

DISCUSSION

This article explores the factors that influence CRC screening, particularly colonoscopy, among rural Appalachian Kentuckians. The results from this study may help to improve our understanding of the unique factors and circumstances that impede or facilitate the adoption of colonoscopy in Appalachian Kentucky. To the authors' knowledge, such insights have not been previously reported.

One of the most intriguing findings from these focus groups was the emphasis on colonoscopy as the predominant or even exclusive screening method for CRC, to the exclusion of other screening modalities. Without prompting by the focus group moderators, colonoscopy emerged as the predominant CRC screening test of interest. Few comments were directed toward any other screening modality. Providers noted that fecal occult blood testing is not considered to be a useful test because any positive result ultimately would need to be resolved with colonoscopy. Most of the providers indicated that they had been trained in flexible sigmoidoscopy and several had performed it in their practices in the past. They no longer provided flexible sigmoidoscopy for 2 reasons: (1) positive findings would require a referral for colonoscopy and (2) reimbursement rates are too low to make providing flexible sigmoidoscopy financially viable for their practices. However, this may not be a limitation in availability of screening because colonoscopy is the preferred endoscopic procedure.

Residents of rural Appalachia provided several important and unique insights regarding their challenges to CRC screening. As previous research has suggested, physician recommendation plays an important role in influencing CRC screening.[13] Although this finding was reinforced by the findings in this study, there were also issues specific to Appalachia that emerged in this regard. Confusion regarding screening recommendations was clearly expressed, as it was not often unclear to patients that their providers recommended screening. This perceived ambiguity translated into a lack of prioritization of colonoscopy by the patients.

Previous research also points to embarrassment and fear as important barriers to colonoscopy from a patient perspective, especially among certain cultural groups. This finding, although evident in this population, is layered with the close-knit community structure that is present in much of rural Appalachia. Concerns about maintaining privacy in these communities is a commonly voiced concern.[18,19] Persons worry that the provider is their friend or neighbor and that their privacy could be compromised by providers or their staff members.

Providers also listed a variety of barriers as reasons for patients not being screened, most of which focused on patient characteristics and the health care delivery system. Consistent with previous qualitative studies of general cancer screening in Appalachia, guidelines were an area of concern for providers.[5,6] Interestingly, few of the barriers providers cited described shortcoming in their own behaviors or practice patterns. Concerns were expressed among health care providers about whether certain procedures and counseling would be reimbursed.[6]

Although there were several areas where providers and patients agreed in their perceptions about CRC screening in rural Appalachian, there were also marked differences in what each group perceived to be the primary barriers to screening.

Both groups expressed a variety of challenges to CRC screening, however, patients, unlike providers cited the most important barriers as those that had to do with the experiences they perceived to be associated with obtaining screening and with health care providers. Both providers and nonproviders emphasized financial concerns as important factors hindering CRC screening. Although patients' financial concerns focused on whether physician practices would be reimbursed (if not, many maintained, they would be reluctant to recommend the screening), the financial concerns expressed by providers focused on the poverty of their patients and low rates of reimbursement. This divergence in financial concerns should prompt discussions between providers and patients regarding reimbursement issues, with providers being careful to clarify the reasons for their recommendations (or lack thereof) for care.

Another important area of divergence involved provider recommendation of CRC screening. Although providers reported that they routinely recommended colonoscopy, patients mentioned a lack of provider recommendation for screening. Although patients reported that they received both oral and written recommendations and reminders to obtain other screening tests such as mammograms, they reported receiving few CRC screening recommendations. This emphasis on other screenings may have led to the assumption by patients that CRC screening is not really necessary. Because receiving physician recommendations is generally viewed as a key influence in the uptake of screening, this inconsistency or even lack of recommendation should be addressed both in enhanced research and clinical practice.[20,21]

Although both patients and providers agreed that CRC screening was a relatively low priority issue in the overall context of health care for this population, the reasons for its lack of importance were slightly different. Both groups agreed that more pressing health concerns often preclude focusing on screening, with patients suggesting that they are not encouraged to be screened for CRC unless they experience symptoms or have a family history of CRC. Providers, on the other hand, reported that they nearly always advised their patients to obtain CRC screening and that in the face of the other more pressing health concerns, patients postponed or neglected CRC screening. Although having pressing health issues is indeed problematic at times, the presentation of persons with multiple morbidities could be seen as an opportunity to advocate for screening because patients are in the health care setting anyway. Providers should take this opportunity to discuss CRC screening and other preventive care measures with patients.

Although many of the challenges to screening reported here apply to other populations, several factors pertain specifically to rural and Appalachian populations such as health care professional shortages, including a lack of accessibility of specialists trained to perform colonoscopy and concerns with privacy and anonymity in small close-knit communities. Researchers and practitioners should be aware of these cultural considerations when developing plans of care and interventions designed to promote CRC screening among this unique population. Future studies should focus on practical solutions to address these issues.

This article also suggests that in rural Appalachia, there are marked differences between the perceptions of health care providers and patients regarding colorectal screening. These areas of agreement and disagreement present both opportunities and challenges for those concerned with increasing screening. Patients and providers seemed to agree that CRC is a salient health issue in Appalachian Kentucky, and screening is an important objective. However, they disagreed regarding a critical issue: the strength and clarity of provider recommendation. Although the provider focus groups indicated that they recommend colonoscopy to their patients, the patient focus groups generally refuted this claim. Previous research on breast cancer screening suggests that clear messages from providers are necessary to increase mammography, and it can be assumed the same applies for other types of cancer screening, such as that for CRC.[22] Practitioners in this area should place special emphasis on discussions regarding CRC screening and be sure that the language being used is consistent with cultural norms. They should also listen carefully for cues from the patients that they are aware of the importance of CRC screening. Involving lay health workers or other community members in messaging may also provide help with this issue.

Finally, the emphasis on colonoscopy as "the" screening test for CRC is problematic in Appalachian Kentucky. The limitation of recommendations to colonoscopy, argu-ably the most expensive and least available screening modality in Appalachian Ken-tucky, raises an important issue requiring additional research: is screening with methods with lower sensitivity better than no screening at all? Or, are the human and financial costs associated with screening using an imperfect test too great to be justifiable?

The authors acknowledge several limitations. First, their sample size and selection approach limits the generalizability of their findings. Second, because data collection took place in rural Appalachian Kentucky, it is unclear whether the results reflect screening influences that are specific to Appalachia or simply to a rural environment. The authors suspect that the confluence of rural and Appalachia fosters additive chal-lenges to obtaining screening. Finally, because medical records were not used, they are unable to verify patients "screening status and providers" claims of having given their patients screening recommendations. Despite these limitations, the authors' results provide among the first published insights on patient and provider perspectives on CRC screening in the highly burdened region of Appalachia.

REFERENCES

1. American Cancer Society. Cancer facts & figures. Alanta: American Cancer Society; 2009.
2. Kentucky Cancer Registry. Age-adjusted cancer mortality rates in Kentucky. 2009. Available at: http://cancer-rates.info/ky/index_mort.php. Accessed June, 2010.
3. Centers for Disease Control. Behavior risk factor surveillance system survey data. 2007. Available at: http://www.cdc.gov/cancer/colorectal/statistics/screeningrates. htm. Accessed September 20, 2008.
4. Centers for Disease Control and Prevention. Screening for colorectal cancer - United States, 1997. MMWR Morb Mortal Wkly Rep 1999;48(6):116–21.
5. Wackerbarth SB, Peters JC, Haist SA. "Do we really need all that equipment?": factors influencing colorectal cancer screening decisions. Qual Health Res 2005;15(4):539–54.
6. Kelly KM, Phillips CM, Jenkins C, et al. Physician and staff perceptions of barriers to colorectal cancer screening in Appalachian Kentucky. Cancer Control 2007; 14(2):167–75.
7. Behringer B, Friedell GH. Appalachia: where place matters in health. Prev Chronic Dis 2006;3(4):A113.
8. Appalachian Regional Commission. Report to the Appalachian Regional Commission. Washington, DC: United States Government Print Office; 1966.
9. Biola H, Pathman DE. Are there enough doctors in my rural community? Percep-tions of the local physician supply. J Rural Health 2009;25(2):115–23.
10. Thompson MJ, Hagopian A, Fordyce M, et al. Do international medical graduates (IMGs) "fill the gap" in rural primary care in the United States? A national study. J Rural Health 2009;25(2):124–34.

11. Basch CE. Focus group interview: an underutilized research technique for improving theory and practice in health education. Health Educ Q 1987;14(4): 411–48.

12. Morgan D. Designing focus group research. In: Stewart M, Tudiver F, Bass MJ, et al, editors. Tools for primary care research. Newbury Park (CA): Sage; 1992. p. 205–30.

13. Sabatino SA, Burns RB, Davis RB, et al. Breast cancer risk and provider recommendation for mammography among recently unscreened women in the United States. J Gen Intern Med 2006;21(4):285–91.

14. Schwandt T. Dictionary of qualitative inquiry. Thousand Oaks (CA): Sage; 2001.

15. Friedemann-Sanchez G, Griffin JM, Partin MR. Gender differences in colorectal cancer screening barriers and information needs. Health Expect 2007;10(2): 148–60.

16. Maxwell J. Qualitative research design: an interactive approach. 2nd edition. Thousand Oaks (CA): Sage; 2005.

17. Strauss AC, Corbin J. Basics of qualitative research: grounded theory procedure and techniques. Thousand Oaks (CA): Sage; 1990.

18. Allan J, Ball P, Alston M. 'You have to face your mistakes in the street': the contextual keys that shape health service access and health workers' experiences in rural areas. Rural Remote Health 2008;8(1):835.

19. Leach CR, Schoenberg NE. The vicious cycle of inadequate early detection: a complementary study on barriers to cervical cancer screening among middle-aged and older women. Prev Chronic Dis 2007;4(4):A95.

20. Ye J, Xu Z, Aladesanmi O. Provider recommendation for colorectal cancer screening: examining the role of patients' socioeconomic status and health insurance. Cancer Epidemiol 2009;33(3–4):207–11.

21. Sarfaty M, Wender R. How to increase colorectal cancer screening rates in practice. CA Cancer J Clin 2007;57(6):354–66.

22. Schueler KM, Chu PW, Smith-Bindman R. Factors associated with mammography utilization: a systematic quantitative review of the literature. J Womens Health (Larchmt) 2008;17(9):1477–98.

Acculturation, Depression, and Function in Individuals Seeking Pain Management in a Predominantly Hispanic Southwestern Border Community

Kristynia M. Robinson, PhD, FNPbc, RN[a],*, Jose J. Monsivais, MD[b]

KEYWORDS

- Acculturation • Chronic pain • Function
- Depression • Hispanic

With the steadily increasing population growth of Hispanics in the United States, especially those of Mexican origin, comes a curiosity of the impact of acculturation on health and illness. The research focus on acculturation has magnified with the conscientious inclusion of minorities in funded research. A database search of Embase, PubMed, and PsychInfo identified more than 17,000 publications using the explosion of search terms "acculturation and Hispanics or Latinos" with two-thirds published between 2001 and 2011. Adding Boolean terms "and health or disease," the overall number in PsychInfo through 2000 fell to 2435, with publications in the past 10 years doubling to more than 5000. In 2005, inclusion of a measure of acculturation was key to receiving funding for this research study.

Acknowledgment of agency support: Funded in part by the National Institutes of Health, National Center on Minority Health and Health Disparities (Grant #P 20 MD000548) A joint venture of The University of Texas at El Paso and The University of Texas Health Science Center at Houston School of Public Health.
The authors have nothing to disclose.
[a] School of Nursing, The University of Texas at El Paso, 1101 North Campbell, El Paso, TX 79902, USA
[b] Hand and Microsurgery Center of El Paso, 10175 Gateway West, #230, El Paso, TX 79925, USA
* Corresponding author.
E-mail address: krobinson@utep.edu

0029-6465/11/$ – see front matter © 2011 Elsevier Inc. All rights reserved.

Acculturation is the process of adapting attitudes, values, customs, beliefs, and behaviors to that of a new and dominant or host culture, that is, the Anglo culture in the United States.[1-4] In studies of the impact of acculturation on health and illness of Hispanics, results are mixed: Acculturation tends to be both protective and deleterious depending on the condition of interest and type of measurement.[5-7] Measurement includes formalized scales, usually language-based,[1] and proxy measures, such as nativity and length of time in the United States.

In general, research related to pain and pain management in the Hispanic population is limited and almost nonexistent when acculturation is added as a research focus. Using PubMed, the authors found two published studies on acculturation and pain—one on cancer pain, the other on orofacial pain. Im and colleagues[8] noted no relationship between cancer pain scores and acculturation level determined by a 5-point Likert scale of preferences related to food, music, customs, language, and friendship. Nevertheless, the proxy measure nativity was correlated with the cancer pain experience: Individuals born outside the United States reported lower pain levels and greater function. Conversely, Riley discovered a relationship between higher levels of orofacial pain and depression and low acculturation as defined by nativity and primary Spanish language use.[9] Although it is known that Hispanics have significantly worse physical health outcomes than Anglos,[10] the role of acculturation in chronic pain is unclear.

As clinicians, it is imperative that we recognize contributing factors, comorbid conditions, and the impact of chronic pain on individuals and families. The purposes of this article are to present evidence that exemplifies the nonsignificant role acculturation plays in expression of pain and function of a predominantly Hispanic population on the United States border; and to identify more meaningful perspectives of culture that may lessen health disparities and improve pain management.

EXEMPLAR STUDY
Background and Significance

Chronic, persistent, or daily recurrent pain is ubiquitous, costly, and disabling, both physically and socially.[11-13] One in 4 Americans suffer from chronic pain, more than twice the number afflicted with diabetes, heart disease, and cancer combined.[14] Yet more than 75% of the time pain is managed inadequately, costing more than $100 billion a year in health care and lost productivity.[15,16]

Pain is a multifaceted syndrome with physiologic and psychosocial contributing factors and expression. Physiologically, pain and depression share common neurologic pathways and affect the same neurotransmitters.[17,18] Individuals with pain often develop depression, and individuals with depression have poorer outcomes when they experience pain.[13]

Culture, health beliefs, and behavior influence health outcomes in this population.[19,20] For example, although Hispanics tend to have worse health outcomes than Anglos,[10] they are at lower risk for depression.[21]

Purpose

Research is limited regarding the role of acculturation in depression and sparse in comorbidity studies of depression and pain. Therefore, the purpose of this exploratory, correlational study was to explore the associations among acculturation, depression, and physical functioning in a predominantly Hispanic population with chronic pain. Sample size was set at 85, based on a priori power analysis to detect a medium effect size of acculturation on pain, function, and depression (α of 0.05 with power of 0.80).[22]

Material and Methods

To protect human rights, the authors observed university policies and procedures related to human subjects, received Institutional Review Board approval from The University of Texas at El Paso prior to data collection, and followed HIPAA (Health Insurance Portability and Accountability Act) regulations to ensure privacy. All data were de-identified and reported in aggregate form, thus maintaining confidentiality and anonymity. Data were collected in 2006 and 2007.

A trained research assistant and clinic staff distributed informed consent forms and surveys in the participants' primary language. Once informed consent was obtained, participants were enrolled in the study. After the completion of the surveys, participants received $5.00 to compensate for their time. The data collection process is described in **Box 1** and measurement in **Table 1**.

Sample and Setting

Through convenience sampling, 92 participants seeking treatment at a specialty clinic with bilingual staff in Texas along the United States/Mexico border were recruited. The specialty clinic is the practice of the second author. All participants received patient-centered care and individualized, multimodal treatment pain management based on best practices. The clinician, blinded to participant status, reviewed the history and conducted a thorough physical examination, and designed a pain management plan in partnership with the patient according to evidence-based practice guidelines.[29]

Analysis

From October through December 2007 data were extracted, coded, cleaned, and imported into a computerized statistical program (SAS version 9.1) for analysis by a university statistician. The statistician calculated descriptive statistics and conducted Pearson correlation coefficients to determine associations among acculturation, depression, and physical functioning using the SAS program and manually calculated z-test for difference between correlations. Post hoc analysis consisted of linear regression, analysis of variance (ANOVA), and multivariate ANOVA.

Box 1
Data collection process

- A bilingual clinic staff member or research assistant recruited patients prior to being seen by the clinician (principal investigator [PI] or co-PI) who was blinded to participation status.

  – Individuals meeting inclusion criteria (English-speaking or Spanish-speaking adults ≥18 years of age requesting treatment of pain who were residents along United States/ Mexico border and able to give informed consent) were asked to participate in the study.

  – Participants were reassured that participation was voluntary and that the decision would not affect the quality of care provided as clinician.

  – Disadvantages and advantages of participation were explained and informed consent was obtained in the patient's primary language.

- Once the consent form was signed, demographic information and scales for pain, acculturation, and functioning were completed in the patient's primary language.

- A bilingual staff member or research assistant reviewed forms for completion. If needed, this trained staff person assisted the individual with completion of the forms.

Table 1
Data collection methods

Variable	Description	Reliability and Validity
Demographic data	Self-reported gender, date and place of birth, marital status, length of time lived in USA	Questions designed specifically for study
Socioeconomic status	Self-reported annual income, occupation, level and place of education (part of demographic data)	
Acculturation	Short Acculturation Scale for Hispanics (SASH) consists of 12 items that tap language use, media preferences, and ethnic social relations. Possible scores range from 12 (low acculturation) to 60 (high acculturation)[23]	Strong internal consistency (coefficient α = 0.92) and validity for Hispanic and non-Hispanic samples[23]
Pain severity	Equidistant 0–10 numerical rating scale (NRS) (from no pain to worst pain possible)[24]	Reported[24]
Depression	Beck Depression Inventory-II (BDI-II) consists of 21 items that measures various symptoms of depression. Possible scores range from 0 to 63, with higher number indicating higher level of depression[25]	High reliability and validity reported for English[25] and Spanish[26] versions
Function	SF-36 short form version 2 (SF-36v2) measures quality of life and overall functioning. It provides 2 summary scores (physical component summary [PCS] and mental component summary [MCS]), and scores for 8 individual scales.[27] Norm-based scoring allows comparison across general and specific adult populations including the elderly.[28] Only the PCS was used for this study	Demonstrated reliability using test-retest and internal consistency methods ($\alpha \geq 0.80$ for subscales and 0.90 for component scores) and content, concurrent, criterion, construct, and predictive validity for English and Spanish versions[28]

Analysis and Results

The sample reflects the general[30] and pain[31,32] population of the Texas community bordering Mexico (**Table 2**). The majority (75%) of participants lived in the United States along the border for 10 years or more; and was Hispanic of Mexican-American origin (79%), married (55%), and female (60%). On average, the sample experienced daily pain levels of 6 with physical functioning below the norm for most Americans,[28] and was mildly depressed, with almost 25% scoring in the moderate to severe range for depression.[28]

The relationship between acculturation and pain level, depression, or function depression was not significant ($P>.05$) even when controlling for socioeconomic status, that is, income and education. Post hoc analysis revealed that gender, nativity

Table 2 Descriptive statistics (n = 92)					
Gender	Age	Ethnicity	BDI	SASH	SF36v2 PCS
55 women (60%)	$\bar{x}$ = 48.8	73 Hispanic (79%)	$\bar{x}$ = 14.5	$\bar{x}$ = 34.5	$\bar{x}$ = 39.8
37 men (40%)	Range 20–83	19 Non-Hispanic (31%)	Range 3–26	Range 20.1–48.9	Range 25.6–53.9

or place of birth (Mexico or United States), and income were correlated to depression and function. These findings are supported by a qualitative project that discovered social roles of women (culture of gender) in this same population to play a significant part in the expression and management of pain. In conclusion, nativity, gender, and income may be more predictive of function and depression in this binational, border population than acculturation.

DISCUSSION

The findings of this study support the conclusion of other scholars and researchers. Acculturation as a descriptor or demographic tells us little about behaviors grounded in individual or group beliefs and attitudes that affect health.[33–36] When acculturation is associated with health behaviors, it does not affect overall health outcomes. For example, Ghaddar and colleagues[37] identified that less acculturated Hispanic Americans ate more fruits and vegetables (not necessarily the daily recommended 5 servings) and were less active then those Hispanics who scored higher in acculturation. However, level of acculturation did not change outcomes in terms of obesity or diabetes.

Acculturation does not inform practice in the acute or primary care setting; nor does it explain ethnic disparities in the recognition and treatment of chronic diseases, particularly chronic pain.[8,9] It is a variable, like gender or ethnicity, that cannot be influenced through nursing or medical practice. As such, it is not useful as a focus for intervention. In an era of globalization, the concept reinforces or maintains stereotyping and the notion that the dominant, namely Anglo, culture is preferred.[2]

Acculturation is a construct beyond its prime. The time has come to move away from this concept toward cultural perspectives of the clinician and the person with pain that do influence health disparities and inform practice. As clinicians, we can provide patient-centered care and incorporate patient beliefs and preferences into clinical decision making.[38] We can identify and measure outcomes in our practice that do make a difference.

On a personal level, living on the border I (K.M.R.) learned Spanish to eliminate the language barrier and promote goodwill with Hispanic patients who prefer to speak Spanish. I find that the more I speak Spanish, the more they speak English; and we can come to a mutually satisfying history, examination, and plan of care. In other instances, I rely on clinicians who are fluent in Spanish to assist me.

REFERENCES

1. Berry JW. Conceptual approaches to acculturation. In: Chun KM, Organista PB, Marín G, editors. Acculturation: advances in theory, measurement, and applied research. Washington, DC: American Psychological Association; 2003. p. 17–37.
2. Abraído-Lanza AF, Armbrister AN, Florez KR, et al. Toward a theory-driven model of acculturation in public health research. Am J Public Health 2006;96(8):1342–6.

3. Negy C, Woods DJ. The importance of acculturation in understanding research with Hispanic-Americans. Hisp J Behav Sci 1992;14(2):224–47. DOI: 10.1177/07399863920142003.

4. Trimble JE. Introduction: social change and acculturation. In: Chun KM, Organista PB, Marín G, editors. Acculturation: advances in theory, measurement, and applied research. Washington, DC: American Psychological Association; 2003. p. 3–13.

5. Carter-Pokras O, Zambrana RE, Yankelvish G, et al. Health status of Mexican-origin persons: do proxy measures of acculturation advance our understanding of health disparities? J Immigr Minor Health 2008;10(6):475–788. DOI: 10.1007/s10903-008-9146-2.

6. Myers HF, Rodriguez N. Acculturation and physical health in racial and ethnic minorities. In: Chun KM, Organista PB, Marín G, editors. Acculturation: advances in theory, measurement, and applied research. Washington, DC: American Psychological Association; 2003. p. 163–86.

7. Organista PB, Organista KC, Kurasaki K. The relationship between acculturation and ethnic minority mental health. In: Chun KM, Organista PB, Marín G, editors. Acculturation: advances in theory, measurement, and applied research. Washington, DC: American Psychological Association; 2003. p. 139–61.

8. Im E, Ho T, Brown A, et al. Acculturation and the cancer pain experience. J Transcult Nurs 2009;20(4):358–70.

9. Riley JL 3rd, Gibson E, Zsembik BA, et al. Acculturation and orofacial pain among Hispanic adults. J Pain 2008;9(8):750–8. DOI: 10.1016/j.jpain.2008.03.007.

10. Woodwell DA, Cherry DA. National ambulatory medical care survey: 2002 summary. Advance data from vital health statistics. Hyattsville (MD): National Center for Health Statistics; 2002. p. 1–44.

11. Singh MK, Patel J, Gallagher RM. Chronic pain syndrome. eMedicine from WebMD. updated May 17, 2010. Available at: http://emedicine.medscape.com/article/310834-overview. Accessed January 20, 2011.

12. Berry PH, Covington EC, Dahl JL, et al. Pain: current understanding of assessment, management, and treatments. Glenview (IL): American Pain Society; 2006. Available at: http://www.ampainsoc.org/ce/enduring/downloads/npc/section_1.pdf. Accessed January 20, 2011.

13. Bair MJ, Robinson RL, Katon W, et al. Depression and pain comorbidity. Arch Intern Med 2003;163:2433–44.

14. American Pain Foundation. Pain facts and figures. Available at: http://www.painfoundation.org/media/resources/pain-facts-figures.html. Accessed January 19, 2011.

15. National Institutes of Health (NIH). NIH guide: new directions in pain research I. 1998. Available at: http://grants.nih.gov/grants/guide/pa-files/PA-98-102.html. Accessed January 19, 2011.

16. National Pain Foundation. Pain in the workplace. 2011. Available at: http://www.nationalpainfoundation.org/articles/894/pain-in-the-workplace?PHPSESSID=5dd55e6608c2cf0e383ea51b4215ca3f. Accessed January 19, 2011.

17. Delgado PL. Common pathways of depression and pain. J Clin Psychiatry 2004;65(Suppl 12):16–9.

18. Schatzberg AF. The relationship of chronic pain and depression. J Clin Psychiatry 2004;65(Suppl 12):3–4.

19. Ponce C, Comer B. Is acculturation in Hispanic health research a flawed concept? JSRI working paper #60. East Lansing (MI): The Julian Samora Research Institute, Michigan State University; 2003.

20. Ruiz P. The role of culture in psychiatric care. Am J Psychiatry 1998;155(12):1763–5.
21. Grant BF, Stinson FS, Haisin S, et al. Immigration and lifetime prevalence of DSM-IV psychiatric disorders among Mexican-Americans and non-Hispanic Whites in the United States. Arch Gen Psychiatry 2004;61(12):1226–33.
22. Cohen J. Quantitative methods in psychology: a power primer. Psychol Bull 1992; 112(1):155–9.
23. Marín G, Sabogal F, Marín BV, et al. Development of a short acculturation scale for Hispanics. Hisp J Behav Sci 1987;9(2):183–205.
24. McQuay HJ, Moore A. Methods of therapeutic trials. In: McMahon SB, Koltzenburg M, editors. Wall and Melzack's textbook of pain. 5th edition. Philadelphia: Elsevier; 2006. p. 416.
25. Beck AT, Steer RA, Brown GK. Manual for the Beck Depression Inventory-II. San Antonio (TX): Psychological Corporation; 1996.
26. Penley JA, Wiebe JS, Nwosu A. Psychometric properties of the Spanish Beck Depression Inventory-II in a medical sample. Psychol Assess 2003;15(4):569–77.
27. Ware JE. SF-36® health survey update. Available at: www.sf-36.org/tools/SF36. shtml. Accessed January 19, 2011.
28. Ware JE, Kosinski M, Dewey JE. How to score version 2 of the SF-36(r) health survey. Lindole (RI): QualityMetric; 2000.
29. Institute for Clinical Systems Improvement (ICSI). Assessment and management of chronic pain. Bloomington (MN): Institute for Clinical Systems Improvement (ICSI); 2005 Nov (revised 2009 Nov). NGC:007602. Available at: http://ngc. gov/content.aspx?id=15525&search=guidelines+for+the+assessment+and+management+of+chronic+pain. Accessed January 20, 2011.
30. FedStats. El Paso MapStats from FedStats. Available at: http://www.fedstats.gov/qf/states/48000.html. Accessed February 22, 2005.
31. Monsivais JJ, Robinson K. Psychological profile and work status of a predominantly Hispanic worker's compensation population with chronic limb pain. Hand (N Y) 2008;3(4):352–8.
32. Monsivais D, McNeill J. Multicultural influences on pain medication attitudes and beliefs in patients with nonmalignant chronic pain syndromes. Pain Manag Nurs 2007;8(2):64–71.
33. Abraído-Lanza AF, Chao MT, Flórez KR. Do healthy behaviors decline with greater acculturation? Implications for the Latino mortality paradox. Soc Sci Med 2005; 61(6):1243–55.
34. Carter-Pokras O, Bethune L. Defining and measuring acculturation: a systematic review of public health studies with Hispanic populations in the United States. A commentary on Thomson and Hoffman-Goetz. Soc Sci Med 2009;69(7):992–5.
35. Hunt LM, Schneider S, Comer B. Should "acculturation" be a variable in health research? A critical review of research on US Hispanics. Soc Sci Med 2004; 59(5):973–86.
36. Zambrana RE, Carter-Pokras O. Role of acculturation research in advancing science and practice in reducing health care disparities among Latinos. Am J Public Health 2010;100(1):18–23 Epub.
37. Ghaddar S, Brown CJ, Pagán JA, Díaz V. Acculturation and healthy lifestyle habits among Hispanics in United States-Mexico border communities. Rev Panam Salud Publica 2010;28(3):190–7.
38. Hulme PA. Cultural considerations in evidence-based practice. J Transcult Nurs 2010;21(3):271–80.

Continuing the Cultural Competency Journey Through Exploration of Knowledge, Attitudes, and Skills with Advanced Practice Psychiatric Nursing Students: An Exemplar

Mary M. Hoke, PhD, RN, PHCNS- BC[a],*,
Leslie K. Robbins, PhD, RN, PMHNP/CNS-BC[b]

KEYWORDS

- Nursing education • Culture competence
- Cultural competency • Hispanic-serving

The provision or the failure to provide culturally competent health care has been shown to influence health outcomes.[1] Numerous cultural competency training and education classes and programs have evolved to address the need for culturally competent health care delivery. The focus of these endeavors has moved from gaining knowledge about specific cultural groups to approaches that integrate attitudes, knowledge, and skills for health care personnel.[1] Attitudes are recognized as the most difficult component to change.[2] Cautions commonly associated with cultural competence education include avoiding stereotyping and using the dominant culture as the norm. Another less frequently articulated criticism is that providers from underrepresented cultural/racial groups, by virtue of their cultural identification, are considered to have cultural competency skills appropriate for interactions with members of

CandyBar Cultures is owned by Dr Mary Hoke.
No other known conflicts of interest exist for the authors.
[a] School of Nursing, MSC 3185, New Mexico State University, PO Box 30001, Las Cruces, NM 88001, USA
[b] School of Nursing, The University of Texas at El Paso, 1101 North Campbell Street, El Paso, TX 79902-0581, USA
* Corresponding author.
E-mail address: mhoke@nmsu.edu

Nurs Clin N Am 46 (2011) 201–205
doi:10.1016/j.cnur.2011.02.004
0029-6465/11/$ – see front matter © 2011 Elsevier Inc. All rights reserved.

their own ethnic/racial group and that these skills are transferable to all cultural groups.[2] Cultural competence has both individual health care provider–client and organizational-policy level implications.[3]

Nursing seeks to provide holistic care that is inclusive of culture considerations. Five major models have generally guided cultural competency nursing education and practice. These include Camphinha-Bacote's *Model of Cultural Competence*, Giger and Davidhizar's *Model of Transcultural Nursing*, Jeffrey's *Cultural Competence*, Leininger's *Cultural Care Diversity and Universality Theory/Model*, Purnell's *Model of Transcultural Health Care*, and Spector's *Health Traditions Model*.[4] There is a growing recognition that nursing educators, who are primarily white, female, and middle-class, have tended to approach cultural competence from a Eurocentric, biomedical perspective. There has been limited acknowledgment of the institutionalized racism in nursing education.[5–7] To counter this limitation/bias, a transformational educational approach that incorporates cultural humility has been recommended.[4,7]

Culture is a broad term that reflects "the totality of socially transmitted behavioral patterns, arts, beliefs, values, customs, lifeways, and all other products of human work and thought, characteristics of a population of people that guide their worldview and decision making."[8(p3)] Cultural identity does not define an individual nor does it mean having exclusive membership in only one group. Rather, cultural identity may encompass membership in a variety of groups simultaneously. Although the concept of cultural competence tends to be connected to intercultural interactions with recognized ethnic /racial minority populations in the United States, it goes much beyond this. For example, cultural identification might be based on sexual identity (heterosexual or homosexual), sensory impairment (hearing or visual), professional discipline (law or nursing), geographic (urban or rural), or generation by age (Baby Boomers or Generation Y), to name just a few.

The purpose of this article is to describe an educational approach used with beginning graduate nursing students to promote their ongoing journey in cultural competency. The approach was incorporated into the graduate community mental health nursing course for students enrolled in the psychiatric mental health (PMH) nurse practitioner (NP) program at a Hispanic-Serving Institution in the American Southwest. The distance education graduate program had an initial 5-day on-campus requirement for the 3-credit community mental health course. In the course component on cultural competence, we were striving to integrate attitudes, knowledge, skill, and cultural humility, but we concentrated our learning objectives on attitudes and cultural humility.

THE STUDENTS

The students in this course were registered nurses (RNs) with a minimum of a baccalaureate in nursing. Their professional experiences varied from acute care to primary care to community care. The amount of professional experience varied from a few months to more than several decades. Student demographic characteristics were also varied in relation to age, ethnicity, gender, sexual identity, disability status (mental and physical), and geographic locations (urban or rural). On average 25% of the class self-identified as being from underrepresented groups.

THE FACULTY

The faculty for the cultural competence component were themselves white women who had experienced a wide variety of health care and academic nursing interactions in which they represented the major or dominant cultural group as well as ones in which they represented the minority or less powerful group. Based on their experiences and education, they thought it was important that the educational component be able to address several important considerations. The curriculum design needed to convey the universality of culture; to recognize that there is as much variety among cultural members as there is between cultural groups; and to convey that doing and using cultural assessments is an important component of high-quality nursing care. From a practical perspective there was a need for a trusting environment in which students were not expected to speak for all members of a cultural group; in which students would not be "put on the spot" for their beliefs and/or past actions; in which students could explore and experience neutral, negative, and positive cultural interactions; and in which they could take risks. Modeling of self-reflection and risk taking by faculty along with the use of adult learning principles would be necessary.

LEARNING OBJECTIVES

At the end of the cultural competence component of the community mental health nursing course, students were expected to demonstrate understanding and respect for one's own and other's cultural beliefs within the health care arena. Specifically objectives included the following:

- Creating a culture using a cultural blueprint that emphasizes concepts important to health;
- Valuing all feelings associated with both the provider and client experiences (including power differentiations and oppression); and
- Valuing the worth and relevance of cultural competence.

PHASE I: FOCUS ON COMPONENTS OF CULTURE AND FEELINGS

Using the CandyBar Cultures[9] proprietary program, Phase I was conducted using small and large groups. Included in this phase were development of an imaginary culture, a simulated health care encounter, and small and large group debriefings. Using a culture blueprint such as those developed by Purnell[8] or Giger and Davidhizar,[10] students working in small groups first developed an imaginary culture and then became immersed in it as they assumed the role of the members of the culture. Cultural assessment models address important aspects that health care professionals would want to understand and consider as they seek to provide culturally competent health care services. Following the development of the imaginary culture, vignettes were assigned to students. For the vignettes, students assumed their assigned character role and incorporated their culture's characteristics as they participated in the role play. Each vignette scenario included a patient, a nurse, and an observer. Also included in the vignette for the patient to assume were presenting symptoms and secondary cultural characteristics known only to the patient. Debriefings occurred at the completion of the health encounter. In small groups, students focused on their feelings and identified examples of culturally neutral, culturally positive, and culturally negative interactions. Following the small group activities, the instructors facilitated a debriefing of the entire class in which key components of cultural competence as viewed by the students were identified.

PHASE II: FOCUS ON CROSS-CULTURAL KNOWLEDGE AND SKILLS

Phase II used a multicultural approach to first provide knowledge updates related to cultural concepts, standards, and research findings. This was followed by education on cross-cultural skills important for PMH NPs. Teaching strategies for this phase included reading assignments, lectures, small group work, and the opportunity to practice skills. Knowledge content addressed cultural assessment and health promotion models, health disparities, cultural and linguistic standards, and rural and border mental health issues. Consistent with Phase I, active learning strategies continued to be used. Included were the use of self-assessment activities to discover unrecognized cultural assumptions and integration of students' professional experiences. In addition, opportunities to explore the incidences and prevalence of mental health disorders, ethnopharmacology, and evidence-based information affecting mental health care delivery were incorporated. The use of cross-cultural skills included the use of cultural assessment instruments, the use of explanatory models to understand the client's view of their illness, use of interpreters, negotiation of provider-client cultural beliefs, active listening, and assessment of organizational cultural competence. Educational strategies used to teach transcultural skills specific to mental health services included case presentations, role playing, and individual reading assignments with discussions.

PHASE III: FOCUS ON INDIVIDUAL SELF-REFLECTION

The final phase sought to extend students' critical reflections through the use of readings and development of a reflection paper. Readings included journal articles and book chapters addressing such topics as sexism, feminism, racism, ageism, white privilege, identity development (racial, ethnic, bicultural), and the culture of oppression. After completion of Phases I and II and the required readings, each individual student submitted a reflection paper. The paper called for students to reflect on interactions occurring with individuals from cultures that were different from their own within their professional nursing practice. Students were required to address 3 areas within the paper. First, using the perspective they brought into the first class session, students reflected on their thoughts and feelings as they related to culture. Next, students reflected on the concepts (attitudes, knowledge, and skills) explored in the class and how these might affect their future professional nursing practice. In the final section, students identified attitudes, knowledge, or skills they believed needed to be improved to facilitate higher levels of cultural competence in their professional nursing interactions. For each identified need, the student developed a professional development plan.

PHASE IV: CULTURAL COMPETENCE PMH CURRICULUM THREAD

Students continued their journey in cultural competence development through the remainder of their graduate work. Cultural competency threads were woven through PMH specialty didactic and clinical courses and were reinforced and evaluated through the use of objective simulated clinical experiences.[11] As a culminating experience, students were required to incorporate culturally competent practice into the planning, implementation, and evaluation of an assigned case study. This provided the students a mechanism to demonstrate cultural humility.

SUMMARY

A recurring comment from students was that the cultural competence component, within the community mental health course, assisted them in becoming more culturally aware, reminded them of how their own culture affects the nursing care they provide, and the need to be open and flexible. Students also shared the view that the debriefing sessions were essential as they sought to integrate insights they discovered during the activities. Students identified active listening, active observing, and being genuine as key components of cultural competency.

This exemplar demonstrates how the use of an integrated approach that addresses knowledge, attitudes, skills, and cultural humility within a graduate PMH NP program can facilitate the ongoing journey of cultural competence development for graduate nursing students. The approach is that which has been recommended in the Institute of Medicine's landmark report *Unequal Treatment: Confronting Racial and Ethnic Disparities in Healthcare*.[1] It builds on the cultural competencies of baccalaureate nursing by strengthening the emphasis on self-awareness, clinical care, and research as recommended by the American Association of Colleges of Nursing.[4]

ACKNOWLEDGMENTS

This work was partially funded by the Division of Nursing, Bureau of Health Professions, Health Resources and Services Administration (Advanced Education Nursing), Department of Health and Human Services under Grant Award # 5D09HP02743-02-00 and title: MENTAL HEALTH IMPROVEMENT VIA NURSING DISTANCE EDUCATION (2004–2007) for $1,091,329.00 The information or content and conclusions are those of the authors and should not be construed as the official position or policy of the funding agency.

REFERENCES

1. Smedley BD, Stith AY, Nelson AR, editors. Unequal treatment: confronting racial and ethnic health disparities. Washington, DC: National Academic Press; 2003.
2. Engebretson J, Mahoney J, Carlson ED. Cultural competence in the era of evidence-based practice. J Prof Nurs 2008;24:172–8.
3. Carpenter-Song EA, Schwallie MN, Longhofer J. Cultural competence reexamined: critique and directions for the future. Psychiatr Serv 2007;58:1362–5.
4. American Association of Colleges of Nursing. Tool kit for cultural competence in master's and doctoral nursing education. Available at: http://www.aacn.nche.edu/education/pdf/Cultural_Competency_Toolkit_Grad.pdf. Accessed January 6, 2011.
5. Duffy ME. A critique of cultural education in nursing. J Adv Nurs 2001;36:487–95.
6. Georges JM. The politics of suffering: implications for nursing science. ANS Adv Nurs Sci 2004;27:250–6.
7. Lancellotti K. Cultural care theory: a framework for expanding awareness of diversity and racism in nursing education. J Prof Nurs 2008;24:179–83.
8. Purnell LD, Paulanka BJ. Transcultural health care: a culturally competent approach. 2nd edition. Philadelphia: FA Davis; 2003.
9. Hoke MM. U.S. Registration No. 3,592,279. Washington, DC: US Patent and Trademark Office; 2009.
10. Giger JN, Davidhizar RE. Transcultural nursing: assessment and intervention. 5th edition. St Louis (MO): Mosby; 2008.
11. Robbins LK, Hoke MM. Using objective structured clinical examinations to meet clinical competence evaluation challenges with distance education students. Perspect Psychiatr Care 2008;44:81–8.

Translation of Family Health History Questions on Cardiovascular Disease and Type 2 Diabetes with Implications for Latina Health and Nursing Practice

Gia T. Mudd, PhD[a],*, Maria C. Martinez, PhD[b]

KEYWORDS

- Family history • Latinas • Cardiovascular disease
- Type 2 diabetes

Recent scientific discoveries have significantly advanced understanding of the role of genetics and genomics in such chronic diseases as cardiovascular disease (CVD) and type 2 diabetes (T2D). Some forms of CVD, such as familial hypercholesterolemia,[1] and T2D, including maturity-onset diabetes of the young,[2] are Mendelian, or single-gene, disorders for which specific risk mutations have been identified. However, CVD and T2D are more commonly multifactorial in nature, resulting from gene-gene and gene-environment interactions.[3,4] Gene variants that increase risk for diseases that are multifactorial have been more difficult to identify, limiting the usefulness of genetic testing for risk assessment. Family history reflects genetic, environmental, and lifestyle influences on health and currently provides the most practical and

This work was funded by an internal grant from the University of Kentucky, Lexington, KY. The translation and evaluation of the Spanish-language family history questions from the Family Healthware tool was conducted as part of a collaborative agreement with the Centers for Disease Control and Prevention.
The authors have nothing to disclose.
[a] College of Nursing, University of Kentucky, Lexington, KY 40536-0232, USA
[b] La Casita Center, 2103 Belmont Road, Louisville, KY 40218, USA
* Corresponding author.
E-mail address: Gia.Mudd@uky.edu

beneficial clinical tool for determining risk for the more common and complex forms of CVD and T2D.[5–8]

Familial patterns of disease suggestive of risk include the presence of multiple affected relatives and early onset of disease.[9] A study of the association of CVD risk with family history by Murabito and colleagues[10] demonstrated that compared with persons without a family history of disease, the odds of developing CVD for persons with a parental history was nearly 1.5 times greater (odds ratio [OR] 1.45; 95% confidence interval [CI], 1.02–2.05) and 2 times greater for persons with a sibling history of disease (OR 1.99; 95% CI, 1.32–3.00). Studies have also demonstrated that a family history of premature coronary heart disease, defined as a coronary event such as myocardial infarction occurring before 55 years of age in a male relative and 65 years of age in a female relative, is associated with increased CVD risk.[11–14] Similar outcomes have been shown in studies of the association of family history with T2D. For example, one study demonstrated that compared with persons with no parental history of T2D, the age-adjusted OR for T2D of persons with maternal or paternal diabetes alone is 3.4 (95% CI: 2.3–4.9) and 3.5 (95% CI: 2.3–5.2), respectively. The OR for offspring of 2 affected parents is 6.1 (95% CI: 2.9–13.0), nearly twice that of persons with 1 affected parent.[15] Results from another study have indicated that T2D risk is positively associated with both the number of affected relatives and degree of relationship.[5]

Owing to the association of familial patterns of disease with increased susceptibility, family history is used to assess risk and guide treatment recommendations. A history of premature coronary heart disease, as defined previously, is considered predictive of individual risk and is used to guide cholesterol prevention and treatment recommendations.[16,17] Family history has also been integrated into global CVD risk scores such as the Reynolds Risk Score[18,19] and QRISK.[20] And familial patterns of T2D are assessed to determine average, moderate, or high risk for disease, dependent on number of and degree of relation to family members with disease.[21]

Because family history elucidates genetic as well as environmental and lifestyle influences on health, it may be of particular value as a clinical tool for screening women of Latino ethnicity, or Latinas. CVD is the leading cause of death of Latinos. The prevalence is higher among women than men, with 34.4% of Latinas affected compared with 31.6% of Latino males.[22,23] T2D is the fifth leading cause of death among Latinos[24] and affects 9.6% of all Latinos 20 years of age and older.[25,26] With an estimated lifetime risk of 52.5%, Latinas are at higher risk for T2D than Latino males, whose risk is 45.4%.[27]

Latinas may experience higher rates of CVD and T2D because of interacting effects of lifestyle behaviors and genetic susceptibility. Studies indicate that Latinas engage in generally low levels of physical activity, have unhealthy dietary practices, and experience high rates of overweight and obesity.[28–30] Genes conferring susceptibility to T2D[31,32] and CVD[33,34] have been identified among Latinos and may interact with lifestyle factors, resulting in higher rates of disease among Latinas.[35,36] Given genetic and lifestyle susceptibilities, family health history screening can provide an important guide for the development of nursing strategies to prevent CVD and T2D among Latinas.

To support the use of family history screening in nursing care of Latina clients, questions from the Centers for Disease Control and Prevention (CDC) Family Healthware tool specific to T2D and CVD were translated from English to Spanish and evaluated using focus group methodology. The translation and evaluation were conducted as part of a pilot study of a community-based intervention to reduce CVD and T2D risk among Latinas. The Family Healthware is a computerized program designed to systematically collect family history information relevant to CVD, stroke, and T2D as well as colorectal, breast, and ovarian cancers.[37] The tool also includes information on individuals' behavioral risk factors, including physical activity, diet, smoking, alcohol use, aspirin use, and current screening history. Using computerized algorithms, the program analyzes data on family history and stratifies risk for each disease as strong, moderate, or average. Tailored health messages are generated that provide information on family history and lifestyle risks accompanied by health promotion recommendations. Details about the development of the Family Healthware, its features, and risk stratification algorithms have been described elsewhere.[37] This article provides a brief report on themes that emerged from focus group discussions during evaluation of the translated family history questions followed by a discussion of the relevance to culturally competent integration of family history information into nursing practice.

METHODS
Sample and Setting

Four focus groups were conducted as part of a formative study to develop a community-based intervention to reduce CVD and T2D risk among Latinas residing in a Midwestern urban area. A purposive sampling strategy was used to ensure representativeness of the local Latina community. Participant eligibility included Latina women who were 18 years of age or older and whose primary language was Spanish. Twenty-one Latinas participated in the formative study, 15 of whom participated in the focus groups. The country of origin of 15 of the participants was Mexico; 6 were from Central or South America. Participants ranged in age from 22 to 65 years with a mean age of 40 years, and approximately half of the women had a high school degree or less.

Procedures

The study was approved by the Institutional Review Board of the University of Kentucky. Each participant was individually consented before initiation of the larger study. During the first session of the larger study, participants completed a sociodemographic form that included information on age, country of origin, language preference, and educational level.

The original English-language version of the Family Healthware tool was translated into Spanish based on guidelines for instrument translation from the World Health Organization,[38] the US Census Bureau,[39] and the Agency for Healthcare Research and Quality.[40] The process included field testing of the translated instrument among Spanish-speaking Latinas using focus group methodology. Focus groups were facilitated by a member of the research team who was a native Spanish speaker. At the beginning of each focus group, a paper-based version of the Spanish translation of questions from the Family Healthware tool specific to CVD and T2D was provided to each participant. Participants were asked to provide feedback on the format, ease of item comprehension and ability to respond, and cultural applicability and acceptability of the family history questions. Each focus group was approximately 2 hours in length. Refreshments were provided during the sessions and participants received a $10 gift certificate as acknowledgment of the value of the information provided and the importance of their expertise to the study.[41,42]

Data Analysis

All focus group sessions were audio taped and recordings were transcribed verbatim. Guided by a process of content analysis used in previous focus group research,[43] 2 investigators on the research team conducted separate analyses of the focus group data. After individually hand-coding transcripts, the investigators jointly reviewed codes and, through a process of consensus, identified emergent themes.

FINDINGS

For the purpose of this article, themes that emerged that can guide use of family history in nursing practice with Latina clients are presented. These can be broadly categorized as: (1) limited knowledge of family health history information; (2) the association of family history and personal health; and (3) communication barriers to the collection and use of family history information in clinical practice.

Limited Knowledge of Family Health History Information

In each of the focus groups, limited knowledge of family health history was identified as a potential barrier to use in clinical practice. As one participant stated, "Sometimes people don't even know about (the health of) their parents." Other participants believed that information on first-degree relatives would not be difficult to ascertain but that people would generally be uninformed as to the health status of second-degree relatives. As explained by one focus group member: "I don't know very much information …about my father's brothers and whether or not they have had (a disease)."

Limited knowledge of detailed information on health conditions was identified by participants as particularly problematic. According to one woman, "…if my father had sugar in the blood, me, what am I going to know about it? I don't have any idea. I only know that he had it and they are asking me to be more specific." The ability to identify the age of disease onset was similarly discussed as presenting difficulty. As explained by one focus group member, "If my father had heart disease, just say a, let's say a heart attack, I don't remember when but I know that he had one. …I don't know if he was sick since his youth or only after a certain age."

Participants expressed concern that limited family health information would result in inaccurate reporting. One woman summarized this by stating, "I like to answer everything because when I don't answer everything I think that (the medical staff) is not going to attend to me. And so you just give whatever response so you don't leave a blank response."

Family Health Information and Personal Health

Another theme emerged regarding the association of the family health history with personal health status. Several focus group members questioned the value of providing family history information, as exemplified by one participant's question: "Why so much about my family if it is my health history?" Another stated, "If I go to the doctor, they don't want to know about all of my family."

There was also discussion regarding the value of providing information on certain family members. Although some participants understood that information on the health of first-degree relatives could have implications for the health of the individual client, the importance of providing health data on more distant family members was not as well understood. As stated by one participant: "I don't see much of a relation to my father's sisters, or the sisters on my father's side, on my mother's side." The relevance of including the health data of relatives who were no longer living was also questioned: "It says relatives or family members living or dead. What does anything have to do with those who have died if, all the same, they are now dead?" A similar concern was the inclusion of information on half-siblings, as exemplified by one woman's question, "And later, here, it says for you to include half-brothers and sisters. Why do they say that? … Why do they put in half-brothers and sisters?"

Participants who recognized the significance of family history relative to personal health status discussed the association of awareness with anxiety. As stated by one woman regarding her awareness of familial patterns of disease, "It worries me because I don't have diabetes; I haven't had a stroke or heart disease. But in making my family tree, I realize that I have this in my family and that I had not considered this." According to one focus group member, the anxiety motivated lifestyle change: "Now that my brother has suffered a stroke… with my history, I am fearful. I have to face this reality and start to take care of myself." Another participant's comment revealed concern that the disclosure of family health information would be interpreted as diagnostic: "If I put that (someone in the family) has diabetes, then they will say that I also have it."

Communication Barriers

Several themes related to communication difficulties that could impede health providers' collection of accurate family history data also emerged from the focus group discussions. A primary concern was that family history terminology would be misunderstood or misinterpreted by clients. For example, reference to "family health history" was unclear to some. As explained by one participant, "But when they say to you 'history,' history has to include everything, how it started, what happened, and how it ended." Variations in terms used to refer to health conditions were also noted to be potentially problematic. As an example, commonly understood terms for "heart attack" were identified as including "stopping of the heart," "heart malfunction," or "infarction." Similarly noted were difficulties related to variable interpretations of the same word, such as "infarction" that is commonly used to refer to either a heart attack or a stroke. Participants also stressed that underlying much of the difficulty with communication were cross-cultural linguistic variations, as summarized by the following comment, "We are a mixed community… Therefore we speak in different ways."

Communication barriers related to the process of provider-client interaction were also emphasized. There was general agreement among participants that responding to direct questioning from health providers was preferable to completing a family history form. As summarized by one participant, "It would be better if the doctor would ask me, 'Your father's history, your mother's, have they had some disease related to the heart, to diabetes?' I think it would be better this way than to fill out all these forms." This was in part because of concern that completing a family history questionnaire immediately before a health care appointment would cause anxiety, as expressed in the following comment from a participant: "…when someone goes to the doctor, they become nervous, especially if they are there to be treated for an illness. And to have to read this while remaining calm, it would not be easy." Also of concern was insufficient provider attention to information solicited on patient health forms. Referring to this, one participant stated, "I never see the doctor or the nurse look at (the information). They just fold it up and put it in a folder."

DISCUSSION

Common themes emerged from the analysis of focus group data with implications for the collection, interpretation, and use of family health information in health care practice. Among these was a general consensus that Latinas would have limited knowledge of the health status of family members. Being uninformed about family health conditions, particularly those of second-degree relatives, and about specific disease information such as age of disease onset, were identified as particular difficulties. Participants were concerned that knowledge limitations would result in inaccurate family history reporting.

In a systematic review on the use of family history in primary care settings, Wilson and colleagues[44] examined studies on the accuracy of self-reported family history and found that people are generally able to correctly report on the absence of disease among family members but not on the presence of disease. Reporting of disease among second-degree relatives and the identification of age of disease onset have boon identified as specific factors that decrease reporting reliability.[45,46] Limited client knowledge of family health information has been noted to be a barrier to physician use of family history in practice.[47,48] Despite the potential disadvantages of self-reported family history, however, this remains the most practical method of data collection in clinical settings.[49]

Although some participants did not understand the importance of collecting family health information, there were indications that focus group members with a family history of CVD and T2D were generally aware of the implications for personal risk. Other studies have reported similar results. For example, a survey of women in a large population-based study on CVD risk awareness demonstrated that those with a family history of CVD were more aware of personal risk than those with no family history.[50] Similarly, the results of a qualitative study on awareness of diabetes risk among Latinos and African Americans suggested that perceived risk was higher among Latinos with a family history of diabetes compared with those without a family history.[51]

The anxiety expressed by focus group members related to awareness of familial patterns of disease has been reported in other studies. Interestingly, the experience of anxiety has been demonstrated to be transitory and not associated with long-term adverse psychological effects.[44] The potential for awareness to support engagement in risk-reducing behaviors, as discussed by participants in the current study, is only partially supported in the literature. Although some researchers have reported more frequent engagement in healthy behaviors among persons with a positive family history of CVD or T2D,[52–54] others have found no association.[55,56] Of most concern are studies in which increased awareness of a positive family history has been negatively associated with health-promoting behaviors,[53,57,58] suggesting that people who attribute disease risk to family history may interpret susceptibility as a nonmodifiable factor and may be less motivated to engage in healthy behaviors.[59]

Several issues related to effective communication arose during the focus group discussions. Primary among these was the need to use language commonly understood among Spanish speakers of various cultural backgrounds. Although much research has been conducted demonstrating the negative effect of client-provider language discordance on clinical outcomes for Spanish-speaking patients,[60–63] little attention has been given the impact of regional Spanish language variations on clinical care.

Reflecting participants' preference to communicate family history information directly to providers, clinicians similarly favor direct patient interview for gathering clients' family health information, noting this can facilitate the collection of more in-depth information.[48] Participants' concern that information communicated by clients was not given sufficient consideration by health professionals has also been addressed in the literature, with clinician time constraints noted to limit attention to the collection and interpretation of family history information, thus decreasing effective use.[64,65]

IMPLICATIONS FOR NURSING PRACTICE

Family history is commonly used in health care practice[66] and the collection and interpretation of family history information has been identified by the National Coalition of Health Professional Education in Genetics (NCHPEG) as a core competency for health professionals.[67] Family history is a particularly effective tool for screening for CVD and T2D risk. Recommendations from both the American Heart Association and the American Diabetes Association underscore the need for health professionals to recognize genetic and behavioral contributions to familial aggregation of CVD and T2D and encourage the collection and use of family history data to guide health care interventions in clinical practice.[17,68,69]

Proficiency in the collection and use of family history information in practice is expected of all nurses. This is reflected in the Consensus Panel on Genetic/Genomic Nursing Competencies.[70] Competent nursing practice includes the ability to elicit a 3-generation family health history and nurses at all levels are expected to critically analyze family history and other relevant genetic and genomic information and to provide appropriate support, education, referral, and advocacy services for clients.[70]

Data from the focus group discussions with Latinas can support competent integration of the collection and use of family history information into nursing practice. Several themes that emerged highlight barriers that have been recognized as relevant to all population groups. For example, clients' limited knowledge of the health status of family members has been identified as a barrier to effective integration of family history into clinical practice across US populations. This has prompted the implementation of public health campaigns to facilitate population-based family health history education.[71] Perhaps the most prominent public health campaign is the US Surgeon General's Family History Initiative.[72] The focus of the campaign is to increase awareness of family history and the implications for personal health risks. The public is encouraged to collect family history information and to share this with other family members as well as with providers to facilitate primary care prevention. Included in the campaign is an online tool, "My Family Health Portrait," available at http://www.hhs.gov/familyhistory, developed to support the collection of family history information. A Spanish-language version is accessible from the Web site that nurses can use to facilitate the collection of family history information with Latinas.

Nursing education of Latina clients on the implications of family history for personal health risk will be integral to minimizing adverse psychological effects and supporting effective risk reduction interventions. An educational resource available to nurses is the toolkit, "Does It Run in the Family?"[73] Developed by the Genetic Alliance in collaboration with community partners, the kit is designed to complement family history tools used in clinical practice. The toolkit is available in English and Spanish at the Genetic Alliance Web site, www.geneticalliance.org/ccfhh. Included are 2 booklets: "A Guide to Family Health History" that educates about the implications of family health history and "A Guide for Understanding Genetics and Health" that provides basic information about genetics and health conditions that run in families.

The current study may also facilitate the development of a Spanish-language version of the CDC's Family Healthware tool that can be used in both clinical and public health settings. The tool would support the collection and analysis of family history data and related lifestyle information. Risk identification and risk-reducing lifestyle recommendations generated by the Family Healthware tool have the potential to guide nursing interventions that address familial and behavioral risk factors.

SUMMARY

CVD and T2D are multifactorial diseases, influenced by genetic, environmental, and behavioral factors and the interactions among these factors. The most effective tool for assessing risk for such complex diseases is the family health history. Reflecting the influences of genes, the environment, and lifestyle behaviors on health, the family history may be a particularly effective screening tool for US Latinas who experience high rates of CVD and T2D likely because of genetic susceptibility interacting with lifestyle factors.

With the increasing integration of family history into clinical practice, nurses are expected to be proficient in the collection of family health history and to provide support, education, referral, and advocacy services for clients based on critical analysis of genetic and genomic information including family history. Themes that emerged from focus groups conducted with Latina participants elucidated potential barriers to the collection and use of family history data in health care.

Several study limitations should be noted, including the small sample size, use of a purposive sampling strategy, and the absence of representation of women of Cuban and Puerto Rican ethnicity. Although the limitations decrease generalizability of the findings, the study provides insight into concerns of Latinas regarding the integration of family history into clinical practice and can support the provision of competent and culturally appropriate nursing care.

REFERENCES

1. Tosi I, Toledo-Leiva P, Neuwirth C, et al. Genetic defects causing familial hypercholesterolaemia: identification of deletions and duplications in the LDL-receptor gene and summary of all mutations found in patients attending the Hammersmith Hospital Lipid Clinic. Atherosclerosis 2007;194(1):102–11.
2. Schober E, Rami B, Grabert M, et al. Phenotypical aspects of maturity-onset diabetes of the young (MODY diabetes) in comparison with type 2 diabetes mellitus (T2DM) in children and adolescents: experience from a large multicentre database. Diabet Med 2009;26(5):466–73.
3. Arnett DK, American Heart Association Writing Group. Summary of the American Heart Association's scientific statement on the relevance of genetics and genomics for prevention and treatment of cardiovascular disease. Arterioscler Thromb Vasc Biol 2007;27(8):1682–6.
4. Prokopenko I, McCarthy MI, Lindgren CM. Type 2 diabetes: new genes, new understanding. Trends Genet 2008;24(12):613–21.
5. Hariri S, Yoon PW, Qureshi N, et al. Family history of type 2 diabetes: a population-based screening tool for prevention? Genet Med 2006;8(2):102–8.
6. Kardia SL, Modell SM, Peyser PA. Family-centered approaches to understanding and preventing coronary heart disease. Am J Prev Med 2003;24(2):143–51.
7. Harrison TA, Hindorff LA, Kim H, et al. Family history of diabetes as a potential public health tool. Am J Prev Med 2003;24(2):152–9.
8. Bennett RL. The family medical history. Prim Care 2004;31(3):479–95.
9. Genetic Red Flags. National Coalition for Health Professional Education in Genetics. Available at: http://www.nchpeg.org/. Accessed November 11, 2010.
10. Murabito JM, Pencina MJ, Nam BH, et al. Sibling cardiovascular disease as a risk factor for cardiovascular disease in middle-aged adults. JAMA 2005;294(24):3117–23.

11. Nasir K, Budoff MJ, Wong ND, et al. Family history of premature coronary heart disease and coronary artery calcification: Multi-Ethnic Study of Atherosclerosis (MESA). Circulation 2007;116(6):619–26.

12. Nasir K, Michos ED, Rumberger JA, et al. Coronary artery calcification and family history of premature coronary heart disease: sibling history is more strongly associated than parental history. Circulation 2004;110(15):2150–6.

13. Wang TJ, Nam BH, D'Agostino RB, et al. Carotid intima-media thickness is associated with premature parental coronary heart disease: the Framingham Heart Study. Circulation 2003;108(5):572–6.

14. de Giorgis T, Giannini C, Scarinci A, et al. Family history of premature cardiovascular disease as a sole and independent risk factor for increased carotid intima-media thickness. J Hypertens 2009;27(4):822–8.

15. Meigs JB, Cupples LA, Wilson PW. Parental transmission of type 2 diabetes: the Framingham Offspring Study. Diabetes 2000;49(12):2201–7.

16. National Cholesterol Education Program Expert Panel on Detection, Evaluation and Treatment of High Blood Cholesterol in Adults. Third report of the National Cholesterol Education Program (NCEP) expert panel on detection, evaluation, and treatment of high blood cholesterol in adults (adult treatment panel III) final report. Circulation 2002;106(25):3143–421.

17. Redberg RF, Benjamin EJ, Bittner V, et al. ACCF/AHA 2009 performance measures for primary prevention of cardiovascular disease in adults: a report of the American College of Cardiology Foundation/American Heart Association task force on performance measures (writing committee to develop performance measures for primary prevention of cardiovascular disease): developed in collaboration with the American Academy of Family Physicians; American Association of Cardiovascular and Pulmonary Rehabilitation; and Preventive Cardiovascular Nurses Association: endorsed by the American College of Preventive Medicine, American College of Sports Medicine, and Society for Women's Health Research. Circulation 2009;120(13):1296–336.

18. Ridker PM, Paynter NP, Rifai N, et al. C-reactive protein and parental history improve global cardiovascular risk prediction: the Reynolds Risk Score for men. Circulation 2008;118(22):2243–51.

19. Bassuk SS. The Reynolds Risk Score—improving cardiovascular risk prediction in women. AAOHN J 2008;56(4):180.

20. Hippisley-Cox J, Coupland C, Vinogradova Y, et al. Derivation and validation of QRISK, a new cardiovascular disease risk score for the United Kingdom: prospective open cohort study. BMJ 2007;335(7611):136.

21. Scheuner MT, Wang SJ, Raffel LJ, et al. Family history: a comprehensive genetic risk assessment method for the chronic conditions of adulthood. Am J Med Genet 1997;71(3):315–24.

22. Rosamond WF, Flegal K, Furie K, et al. Heart disease and stroke statistics—2008 update: a report from the American Heart Association Statistics Committee and Stroke Statistics Subcommittee. Circulation 2008;117(4):e25–146.

23. Hunt KJ, Resendez RG, Williams K, et al. All-cause and cardiovascular mortality among Mexican-American and non-Hispanic White older participants in the San Antonio Heart Study— evidence against the "Hispanic paradox". Am J Epidemiol 2003;158(11):1048–57.

24. Heron M. Deaths: leading causes for 2004. Natl Vital Stat Rep 2007;56(5):1–95.

25. Office of Minority Health & Health Disparities. Eliminate disparities in diabetes. 2008. Available at: http://www.cdc.gov/omhd/AMH/factsheets/diabetes.htm. Accessed April 4, 2008.

26. National Institute of Diabetes and Digestive and Kidney Diseases. National diabetes statistics. NIH Publication: No. 06–3892; 2005. Available at: http://diabetes.niddk.nih.gov/dm/pubs/statistics/#7. Accessed February 18, 2008.

27. Narayan KM, Boyle JP, Thompson TJ, et al. Lifetime risk for diabetes mellitus in the United States. JAMA 2003;290(14):1884–90.

28. Centers for Disease Control and Prevention. Prevalence of fruit and vegetable consumption and physical activity by race/ethnicity—United States, 2005. MMWR Morb Mortal Wkly Rep 2007;56(13):301–4.

29. Keller C, Fleury J. Factors related to physical activity in Hispanic women. J Cardiovasc Nurs 2006;21(2):142–5.

30. Murtaugh MA, Herrick JS, Sweeney C, et al. Diet composition and risk of overweight and obesity in women living in the southwestern United States. J Am Diet Assoc 2007;107(8):1311–21.

31. Palmer ND, Lehtinen AB, Langefeld CD, et al. Association of TCF7L2 gene polymorphisms with reduced acute insulin response in Hispanic Americans. J Clin Endocrinol Metab 2008;93(1):304–9.

32. Duggirala R, Blangero J, Almasy L, et al. Linkage of type 2 diabetes mellitus and of age at onset to a genetic location on chromosome 10q in Mexican Americans. Am J Hum Genet 1999;64(4):1127–40.

33. Crawford DC, Sanders CL, Qin X, et al. Genetic variation is associated with C-reactive protein levels in the Third National Health and Nutrition Examination Survey. Circulation 2006;114(23):2458–65.

34. Chiu L, Hamman RF, Kamboh MI. Apolipoprotein A polymorphisms and plasma lipoprotein(a) concentrations in non-Hispanic Whites and Hispanics. Hum Biol 2000;72(5):821–35.

35. Hsu YH, Niu T, Song Y, et al. Genetic variants in the UCP2-UCP3 gene cluster and risk of diabetes in the Women's Health Initiative Observational Study. Diabetes 2008;57(4):1101–7.

36. Scuteri A, Sanna S, Chen WM, et al. Genome-wide association scan shows genetic variants in the FTO gene are associated with obesity-related traits. PLoS Genet 2007;3(7):e115.

37. Yoon PW, Scheuner MT, Jorgensen C, et al. Developing Family Healthware, a family history screening tool to prevent common chronic diseases. Prev Chronic Dis 2009;6(1):A33.

38. World Health Organization (n.d.). Process of translation and adaptation of instruments. Available at: http://www.who.int/substance_abuse/research_tools/translation/en/. Accessed March 15, 2008.

39. U.S. Census Bureau (2006). "Census bureau guideline: Language translation of data collection instruments and supporting materials. Available at: http://www.census.gov/cac/2010_census_advisory_committee/language_translation_guidelines.html. Accessed January 28, 2008.

40. CAHPS II Cultural Comparability Team (2006). Guidelines for Translating CAHPS Surveys. Available at: https://www.cahps.ahrq.gov/content/resources/pdf/Guidelines_Translation.pdf. Accessed January 21, 2008.

41. Singer E, Kulka RA. Paying respondents for survey participation. In: Ver Ploeg M, Moffitt RA, Citro CF, editors. Studies of welfare populations: data collection and research issues. Washington, DC: Committee on National Statistics; 2002. Available at: http://aspe.hhs.gov/hsp/welf-res-data-issues02. Accessed February 18, 2007.

42. Grady C. Payment of clinical research subjects. J Clin Invest 2005;115(7):1681–7.

43. Frazier L, Calvin AO, Mudd GT, et al. Understanding of genetics among older adults. J Nurs Scholarsh 2006;38(2):126–32.

44. Wilson BJ, Qureshi N, Santaguida P, et al. Systematic review: family history in risk assessment for common diseases. Ann Intern Med 2009;151(12):878–85.

45. O'Neill SM, Rubinstein WS, Wang C, et al. Familial risk for common diseases in primary care: the Family Healthware impact trial. Am J Prev Med 2009;36(6): 506–14.

46. Murabito JM, Nam B-H, D'Agostino RB, et al. Accuracy of offspring reports of parental cardiovascular disease history: the Framingham Offspring Study. Ann Intern Med 2004;140(6):434–40.

47. Flynn BS, Wood ME, Ashikaga T, et al. Primary care physicians' use of family history for cancer risk assessment. BMC Fam Pract 2010;11(45). Available at: http://www.biomedcentral.com/1471-2296/11/45. Accessed November 11, 2010.

48. Wood ME, Stockdale A, Flynn BS. Interviews with primary care physicians regarding taking and interpreting the cancer family history. Fam Pract 2008; 25(5):334–40.

49. Sivapalaratnam S, Boekholdt SM, Trip MD, et al. Family history of premature coronary heart disease and risk prediction in the EPIC-Norfolk prospective population study. Heart 2010;96(24):1985–9.

50. Mosca L, Mochari H, Christian A, et al. National study of women's awareness, preventive action, and barriers to cardiovascular health. Circulation 2006; 113(4):525–34.

51. Cullen KW, Buzek BB. Knowledge about type 2 diabetes risk and prevention of African-American and Hispanic adults and adolescents with family history of type 2 diabetes. Diabetes Educ 2009;35(5):836–42.

52. Winnicki M, Somers VK, Dorigatti F, et al. Lifestyle, family history and progression of hypertension. J Hypertens 2006;24(8):1479–87.

53. Thanavaro JL, Moore SM, Anthony M, et al. Predictors of health promotion behavior in women without prior history of coronary heart disease. Appl Nurs Res 2006;19(3):149–55.

54. Baptiste-Roberts K, Gary TL, Beckles GL, et al. Family history of diabetes, awareness of risk factors, and health behaviors among African Americans. Am J Public Health 2007;97(5):907–12.

55. LeBlanc KE, Scarinci IC, LeBlanc LL, et al. Modifiable high-risk behaviors for cardiovascular disease among family physicians in the United States. A national survey. Arch Fam Med 1997;6(3):246–50.

56. Kip KE, McCreath HE, Roseman JM, et al. Absence of risk factor change in young adults after family heart attack or stroke: the CARDIA study. Am J Prev Med 2002; 22(4):258–66.

57. Walter FM, Emery J. Perceptions of family history across common diseases: a qualitative study in primary care. Fam Pract 2006;23(4):472–80.

58. Runions S, Arnaert A, Sourial R. Causal attributions and health behavior choices among stroke and transient ischemic attack survivors. J Neurosci Nurs 2006;38-(Suppl 4):288–95.

59. Murphy B, Worcester M, Higgins R, et al. Causal attributions for coronary heart disease among female cardiac patients. J Cardiopulm Rehabil 2005;25(3): 135–43.

60. Fernandez A, Schillinger D, Grumbach K, et al. Physician language ability and cultural competence. An exploratory study of communication with Spanish-speaking patients. J Gen Intern Med 2004;19(2):167–74.

61. Flores G, Laws MB, Mayo SJ, et al. Errors in medical interpretation and their potential clinical consequences in pediatric encounters. Pediatrics 2003;111(1): 6–14.

62. Sudore RL, Landefeld CS, Perez-Stable EJ, et al. Unraveling the relationship between literacy, language proficiency, and patient-physician communication. Patient Educ Couns 2009;75(3):398–402.

63. Sudore RL, Landefeld CS, Karliner LS, et al. Do professional interpreters improve clinical care for patients with limited English proficiency? A systematic review of the literature. Health Serv Res 2007;42(2):727–54.

64. Yoon P, Scheuner M. The family history public health initiative. In: Centers for Disease Control and Prevention Office of Genomics and Disease Prevention, ed., Genomics and population health: United States 2003. Atlanta (GA); 2004. Available at: http://www.cdc.gov/genomics/about/reports/2003/chap06.htm. Accessed February 12, 2007:39-45.

65. Wattendorf DJ, Hadley DW. Family history: the three-generation pedigree. Am Fam Physician 2005;72(3):441–8.

66. Berg AO, Baird MA, Botkin JR, et al. National Institutes of Health state-of-the-science conference statement: family history and improving health. Ann Intern Med 2009;151(12):872–7.

67. National Coalition for Health Professional Education in Genetics. Core competencies in genetics essential for health professionals (2007), 3rd edition Lutherville (MD): 2007. Available at: http://www.nchpeg.org/index.php?option=com_content&view=article&id=107&Itemid=84. Accessed November 11, 2008.

68. Pearson TA, Blair SN, Daniels SR, et al. AHA Guidelines for primary prevention of cardiovascular disease and stroke: 2002 update: consensus panel guide to comprehensive risk reduction for adult patients without coronary or other atherosclerotic vascular diseases. American Heart Association Science Advisory and Coordinating Committee. Circulation 2002;106(3):388–91.

69. American Diabetes A. Standards of medical care in diabetes-2010. Diabetes Care 2010;33(Suppl 1):S11–61.

70. Consensus Panel on Genetic/Genomic Nursing Competencies. Essentials of genetic and genomic nursing: competencies, curricula guidelines, and outcome indicators. 2nd edition. Silver Spring (MD): American Nurses Association; 2009.

71. Yoon P, Scheuner M, Gwinn M, et al. Awareness of family health history as a risk factor for disease—United States, 2004. MMWR Morb Mortal Wkly Rep 2004; 53(44):1044–7.

72. US Department of Health and Human Services Office of the Surgeon General. Surgeon general's family health history initiative 2004. Available at: http://www.hhs.gov/familyhistory/. Accessed November 1, 2010.

73. Edelson V, Terry S, O'Leary J, et al. Community centered family health history. Collaboration across communities: how do you make research community-specific and universally-relevant? Genetic Alliance Monograph Series 2010;4. Available at: http://www.geneticalliance.org/sites/default/files/ksc_assets/publications/ccfhh_monograph_final.pdf. Accessed November 11, 2010.

Cultural Competency: Beyond the Vital Signs. Delivering Holistic Care to African Americans

Linda D. Wilson, PhD, MSN, CNS

KEYWORDS

- Cultural competence • African Americans • Health disparities
- Cultural knowledge • Cultural assessment

Factors such as changing demographics, an aging population, escalating unemployment, increasing underinsured or uninsured, and the growing nursing shortage have greatly impacted health care outcomes and contributed to health disparities in this country.[1] Healthy People 2020 goals of promoting health and preventing diseases are aimed at eliminating health disparities.[2] Inevitably, these disparities are influenced by race and ethnicity.[3,4] Nurses must develop a cultural awareness and a deeper appreciation and respect for the rights of all individuals. However, when cultural beliefs and practices are not appropriately assessed and acknowledged, patient behaviors may be perplexing to nurses and result in delivery of inappropriate care. Therefore, nurses must go beyond just assessing vital signs to improve health outcomes for all. Cultural competency is fundamental to bridging the gap between inadequate care and optimal holistic health care. When cultural differences are ignored, barriers to effective health serves may emerge.

The United States Department of Health & Human Services, Office of Minority Health identifies culturally competent nursing as "a cornerstone of caring," and suggests practitioners ask the following questions of themselves: "Have you ever experienced a situation where you were unsure about the best way to approach a patient and family because of [cultural], racial or ethnic concerns? Was there ever a time when language, [cultural or ethnic] differences prevented you from effectively communicating with a patient [or the family]"?[5]

Nurses often consider these questions when working with patients from other countries. However, language barriers such as dialect, or cultural and religious beliefs can

The author has nothing to disclose.
MTSU School of Nursing, Middle Tennessee State University, Cason-Kennedy Nursing Building Office 225, Murfreesboro, TN 37132, USA
E-mail address: lcovingt@mtsu.edu

sometimes adversely impact nurses' ability to work with patients from different racial and or ethnic backgrounds within the American culture. Cultural dissonance may cause misunderstanding and compliance issues, which can negatively influence health outcomes, and this can be particularly true for those in the African American community.

Unless nurses provide culturally competent care, the outcome may be less than optimal. Incongruencies and misunderstandings can lead to misdiagnoses, further contributing to the health disparities in this country. Individuals from some cultures may not behave the way the nursing culture expects. When this occurs, the choices are to provide substandard nursing care or make changes to provide optimal holistic care.

Health care spending in the United States accounts for more than 17% of the nation's gross domestic product (GDP). In 2010, more than $1107 billion were spent on health care, and this number is expected to surpass $1507 billion by 2015.[6] United States health care spending is among the highest of all industrialized countries. As the population diversity increases, more ethnic minorities will enter the health care system sicker, with chronic illnesses, and a tendency to use emergency rooms as the primary source of heath care. The health care cost for chronic disease treatment is estimated to account for more than 75% of the national health expenditures,[7] and this cost is expected to increase dramatically.

Research supports a direct relationship between inequality and negative health outcomes. Race and ethnicity are associated with inequality in health care access, and negative health outcomes. Eliminating these disparities has become a national priority. The Patient Protection and Affordable Care Act was signed into law in March of 2010. This new health reform law has the goal of reducing disparities through making the health system more accessible for most Americans by 2014. However, access is only one barrier to health care. Other dynamics, such as cultural and religious beliefs and historical experiences, greatly impact health care outcomes for African Americans.

The manner in which nurses care for patients and their responses to this care, and definitions of health, illness, disease, and their causes are all greatly influenced by culture. Therefore, nurses must possess the ability and knowledge to communicate and understand health behaviors that are rooted in culture. Having this ability and knowledge can help eliminate barriers. Nurses must not only be cognizant of potential barriers but also participate in developing policies, practices, and procedures to deliver culturally competent care.

Nurses are mandated to go beyond the vital signs to provide culturally competent care. Cultural competence includes the ability to work effectively across cultures in a way that acknowledges and respects the culture of the other person. According to the U.S. Department of Health & Human Services,[2] a culturally competent health care provider is one who delivers effective clinical care based on knowledge and skills of a specific racial or ethnic group. To provide appropriate care, the nurse should understand how cultural values influence patients and families response to the health care provider.[8]

Developing cultural competency is an ongoing process, one that involves evaluating, adapting, and reevaluating. For nurses, cultural competence is a test of their ability to truly care for patients; it is going beyond vital signs to not only implement proficient clinical skills but also provide optimal holistic care.

DEMOGRAPHIC TRENDS AND NURSING

With more than 3 million members, the nursing profession is the largest segment of the health care workforce. With the increasing minority population and decreasing minority representation in nursing, the American Academy of Nursing Expert Panel on Culturally Competent Nursing Care[9] stated that nurses, as the largest workforce in the health care system, have the greatest potential to impact changes related to inequities in accessibility to health care. Nurses spend more time in direct patient care than any other group of health care providers and work in a variety of settings.[10] Therefore, nurses have a unique opportunity to help improve access to care, quality of care, and health outcomes for patients, especially those subject to racial and ethnic health disparities.[11]

Projections for 2010 indicate that more than 28% of the United States population will be represented by an ethnic-minority culture; 13.5% of the population identify themselves as African Americans, and this number is estimated to be 40.2 million in the 2010 census.[12,13] As ethnic minority populations increase, African American patients entering the health care system will mirror this change. Without appropriate adjustments in attitudes, beliefs, and structures in the health care system, a growing disparity in health outcomes will persist.[14] The American Nurses Association position statement,[15] American Academy of Nursing Expert Panel on Cultural Competency,[9] and National League of Nursing's Public Policy Agenda 2009–2010[10] all identified a link between cultural competence education and reducing health care disparities, and have subsequently enacted programs to increase minority representation in nursing, because it is believed that more ethnic minority nurses will help reduce health care disparities.[9,10,15] Meanwhile, ethnic and racial disparities between the population and health care providers continue to widen.

As the changes in demographics persist, a shortage of more than 480,000 nurses by 2020 is estimated. This shortage will be more apparent for ethnic-minority nurses. African Americans will account for 4.2% of the nursing profession, and will constitute 13% of the population.[16] According to Eisner and Ellis,[17] increasing minority representation in the health workforce will improve health care delivery. Minority health professionals express a greater propensity to practice in underserved areas compared with nonminorities. Health professionals who share the same culture and language with the patients they serve are believed to be able to provide more effective care.[17] Because it is unlikely in the foreseeable future that most ethnic minority patients will be treated by racially concordant nurses, given the differing ratio of patient and nurse demographics, most African Americans will be cared for by non–African American health care providers. Therefore, providers must be culturally competent.[17] Nurses, regardless of ethnicity, should want to be culturally competent to understand, communicate with, and effectively interact with their patients. By doing so, nurses can be pivotal in reducing health care disparities.

If health care consumption patterns remained constant over time, the increase demand for full-time-equivalent registered nurses per thousand population would increase from 7 to 7.5 in 2020.[18,19] The literature suggests that ethnic minorities have different patterns of health care use from whites. Inequality in access to care accounts for some of these differences. Nurses can play a crucial role in increasing minority use of the health care system by providing culturally competent care. African American nurses have a greater propensity to practice in urban and underserved areas than nonminority nurses. However, as the number of minority nurses decreases and the ethnic minority population increases, nurses of all ethnic backgrounds will need to provide culturally competent care to reduce health disparities.

THE AFRICAN AMERICAN EXPERIENCE

Providing culturally competent care is multidimensional, including aspects of previous health/illness experiences, religious and cultural beliefs, and environmental and historical facets of care.[3,20] Health and illness are uniquely defined and grounded in a person's own culture, particularly for African Americans because historical and religious factors have greatly impacted the nurse–patient relationship.

Health equity is the state of a population's health that occurs when no inequalities exist in access to and receipt of health information, prevention and treatment services, and end of life care. According to Stacks and colleagues,[21] a direct correlation exists between inequality and negative health outcomes. Of all population groups in the United States, African Americans experience the greatest inequalities in overall cancer incidence and mortality.[22] Health disparities in the African American community are well documented for heart disease, HIV/AIDS, type 2 diabetes, asthma, infant mortality, and even life expectancy and cancer.[20,22–25]

Demographic trends and health disparities require a transformation for nurses to be prepared to meet the health needs of African Americans, and all patients. The government's initiative for health care providers to become culturally competent has prompted an increased awareness of this issue. Consequently, Healthy People 2020[26] challenges health care professionals to take steps to ensure that good health and long life are enjoyed by all.

Not everyone is comfortable with traditional Western medicine. Being colorblind and ethnocentric (ie, saying that everyone is alike, and the American way is the best or only way) will not address the health care needs of all Americans, especially African Americans. To change health outcomes, historical and religious experiences must be considered when working with African Americans.

CULTURE AND CULTURAL COMPETENCE

Culture influences how people perceive, believe, and evaluate their lived experiences. Actions and decisions are governed by culture, which guides thoughts, feelings, being, and how we behave in society.[15] Culture is transmitted across generations and is a support for survival in a specific environment. Domains such as family roles, health care practices, religion, and communication are essential attributes that define an individual's culture. Culture shapes values, knowledge, customs, emotions, rituals, traditions, and norms, which are embedded in behaviors.[27] Mistrust and hostility toward Western traditional health care are entrenched in the culture of African Americans because of centuries of discrimination and unethical research practices. Cumulative effects of negative clinical research experiences, of which Tuskegee is only the best known, continue to foster distrust of health care providers and the health care system within the African American community.[28,29] Managing historical hostility starts with recognizing the uniqueness and historical oppression of African Americans as a part of their culture. Although everyone deserves culturally congruent care, it must be specific to patterns of reaction and reality.

Cultural competence requires an egalitarian relationship among the nurse, patient, and patient's family. It decreases the potential for assumed similarity, which implies that all people share the same beliefs.[15] A considerable amount of literature explores the issue of cultural competence, and strongly supports the fact that health professionals can provide more effective and efficient services if they are knowledgeable and sensitive to the cultural backgrounds of their patients.[20,24,25,27]

Cultural competence should be a priority in nursing practice, given the current and projected United States demographics and health disparities in people of diverse racial, ethnic, and cultural backgrounds. As a major contributor to reducing the gap in health care disparities, cultural competence promotes the delivery of care in a respectful manner predicated on cultural beliefs, practices, and needs. The goal of cultural competence is to achieve equal and quality health care outcomes.[18,20,21,26]

A corresponding change in behavior is required with cultural competence, unlike earlier ideas of cultural sensitivity and awareness that were often embraced with no corresponding adjustment in behavior. Achieving cultural competence is multifaceted, especially with African Americans, because the "Black experience" in this country is vastly different from that of other immigrants.[20,30,31] Providing care that incorporates awareness of cultural influences can help reduce the gap in health disparities for African Americans.

Barriers to Cultural Competence

Many challenges related to providing culturally competent care have been identified, including recognizing clinical differences among ethnic and racial groups (ie, higher risk of hypertension and renal failure in African Americans) and communication.[20,24,25] Trust or mistrust, as most researchers describe it, and for good reason, is a significant challenge to providing culturally competent care in the African American community. For some patients, authority figures are immediately mistrusted. Historical relationships with authority make many people as suspicious of the caregivers themselves as they are of the care. Byrd[32] and others[20,27] noted the reluctance of African American to seek traditional health care relates to a negative history with Western medicine and considerable disillusionment with unethical research practices. However, this mistrust dates as far back as the early 1600s when Africans were forcibly brought to this country as slaves. Unlike any other ethnic group, the African American experience has been one of dehumanization.[20]

CULTURAL COMPETENCE THEORIES OF CARE FOR AFRICAN AMERICANS

Several theories and assessment tools on cultural diversity have been developed and revised over the past 40 years, including Leininger's Transcultural Model,[33–35] Campinha-Bacote's Culturally Competent Model of Care/Process of Cultural Competence in the Delivery of Healthcare Services,[36–38] Geiger and Davidhizer's Transcultural Assessment Model,[27,39] and Andrew and Boyle's Transcultural Concepts in Nursing Care.[24]

One model in particular, the Process of Cultural Competence in the Delivery of Healthcare Services,[20] has been frequently used to promote cultural competence with African American patients. Cultural competence is a "process in which the nurse continuously strives to achieve the ability and availability to effectively work within the cultural context of a client [individual, family, community]."[20] According to Campinha-Bacote,[19,36] cultural competence is a journey, not a destination, in which not only must differences be recognized but also similarities must be built upon.

The integration of five constructs form the foundation of the practice model by Campinha-Bacote: cultural desire, cultural awareness, cultural knowledge, cultural skill, and cultural encounters.[20,36–38] This model asserts that health care professionals begin their journey toward becoming culturally competent by addressing overt and covert barriers to care; assessing the level of awareness and sensitivity toward African American patients; conducting a cultural assessment; obtaining knowledge about this cultural group; and maintaining effective clinical encounters.

According to Campinha-Bacote,[36] barriers are defined as real or perceived gaps to providing quality care that are compounded by the relationship that health and illness has to ethnicity. These barriers include African American mistrust of the health care system, access to care issues, stigmas related to diseases that disproportionately affect African Americans, support systems, and bias in medical decision making.

CULTURAL DESIRE

Cultural desire involves commitment, motivation, compassion, authenticity, humility, openness, availability, and flexibility. One must want to be engaged in the process of cultural competence, regardless of cross-cultural conflict, and have a passion for caring. Campinha-Bacote[20,36] asserts that cultural desire is when a nurse "wants" to be involved in providing culturally competent care, not when one is "required" to do so. Cultural desire is the cornerstone of cultural competence. It allows for authenticity and a truthfulness of wanting to learn about others. Cultural desire begins with wanting to treat others with humility, respect, dignity, and justice. "Human dignity is required for social justice which is vital to achieve equality in health outcomes. Because of the correlation between inequality and negative health outcomes, nurses must consciously connect cultural competence with social justice."[20]

CULTURAL AWARENESS

Cultural awareness is the next step toward cultural competency, which involves an understanding of how one's own culture influences the way one thinks and acts. It is self-examination of one's own prejudices and biases toward other cultures. Cultural awareness is a deliberate process of becoming cognizant of one's own beliefs through an in-depth exploration of self, while being sensitive to the worldviews of others. Self-awareness allows for a conscious awakening to racial and ethical injustices in the health care system and reveals the power imbalances in the patient–nurse relationship in effort to develop a mutually beneficial partnership.[36] The importance of this construct is to prevent the health care professional from engaging in the phenomena of cultural imposition—the tendency to impose one's values on another culture[35]—and to prevent unequal treatment because of personal beliefs and biases.

Before one can begin to understand another's culture, one must understand self first. Personal biases can lead to unequal treatment and misdiagnosis. For instance, more African American are misdiagnosed or overdiagnosed with psychiatric disorders, resulting in inaccurate treatment or overtreatment with antipsychotic drugs.[40] Cultural awareness allows for understanding and determination of where one is along the continuum from unconscious to conscious competence. Unconscious incompetence is when a health care professional is not aware that cultural differences exist. Further along the continuum is conscious incompetence, when health care professionals still do not understand another's culture but are aware of this lack of understanding and that differences exist. Cultural awareness allows for nurses to "examine if racism exists in health care and the role it plays in health disparities."[20]

CULTURAL KNOWLEDGE

Cultural knowledge is an educational process that allows one to obtain information about diverse worldviews. The meaning of health/illness, impact of religion on health/illness, historical experiences, disease incidence/prevalence, and biologic and drug metabolism variations are essential for nurses to know to provide culturally competent care for African Americans.[20] Cultural knowledge prevents the assumption that all individuals are the same within a specific group. Meanwhile, nurses must be conscious of the dynamics inherent when cultures interact. Individuals often misjudge other's actions based on learned expectations and culturally prescribed patterns of communication and decision-making skills. Without cultural knowledge, misinterpretations or misjudgments may emerge.

A conscious effort is required for health care professionals to become knowledgeable about cultural differences. For example, in the African American culture, pain is frequently perceived as inevitable, whereas illness is believed to be of natural causes such as impurities, or unnatural forces such as punishment from God.[27] Traditionally, it was believed that body parts should remain intact as much as possible. Therefore, organ donation is not an option for some African Americans. Without knowledge of this cultural implication, behavior related to organ donations is perplexing to many in the health care system, especially as organ donation and transplantation disparities widen in this country.

Many African Americans mistrust and are suspicious of doctors and nurses, and therefore they seek traditional health care as a last resort. Instead, home or natural remedies are used to treat illness, and spiritual advisors serve as health care providers, particularly for elderly African Americans. Seeking an herbalist and folk medicine for remedies has been a tradition for years, partly because of the lack of access to health care. Folk medicine tends to center on magical aspects of illnesses, such as hexes, roots, and divine displeasure of people or their offspring. This spiritual–magical schema oftentimes views the allopathic physician as inferior to an evangelist who is believed to be spiritually gifted in the healing arts.[17,33]

When attaining cultural knowledge, religion is very important to address because it directs health care practices, often conflicting with traditional health care.[41,42] Health is believed to be a gift from God, whereas illness is a separation from God or the work of the devil. Faith in God is a major inner strength. Spiritual leaders are highly respected. Many believe that ministers, folk healers, and psychics have the ability to predict and possibly prevent death.[24,42,43] Religion is perceived as a source of emotional support and in many ways correlates with improved health outcomes.

The challenge in realizing improved health outcomes among African Americans is to maximize the positive influences of faith while minimizing the negative ones. Occasionally, belief in God may be accompanied by a reduction in medication compliance, thus complicating health care by delaying appropriate interventions.[43] A fundamentalist religious belief is that God will cure illness without medical treatment, with the concurrent belief that roots or spells will cause or cure cancer. These beliefs often increase the likelihood of a patient presenting with late stages of cancer. Research indicated that African American women who believed in God as a controlling agent over health were less likely to obtain mammography and clinical breast examination.[44,45] According to Polzer and Miles,[46] strong spirituality in African American patients with diabetes correlated with self-management of the disease and greater noncompliance with a diabetic regimen.

Knowledge of biologic and drug metabolism variations is essential for cultural competence. The basic challenge of recognizing clinical differences among people of ethnic and racial groups is strongly supported in the literature. African Americans have a higher incidence of chronic illness, a higher mortality rate, and poorer health outcomes. Many of the chronic diseases have a genetic component, such as sickle cell anemia, asthma, and hypertension. The causes of these inequalities are complex and believed to reflect social and economic disparities, such as inequalities in work, income, education, and overall standard of living; barriers to high-quality health care; and racial discrimination, more so than biologic differences associated with race.[11,18,23,47,48]

Underwood and colleagues[49] contend that African Americans are overburdened with diseases, contributing to the disparities in health care. Among the disease-specific examples of racial and ethnic disparities in the United States is the cancer incidence among African Americans. Although the overall racial disparity in cancer death rates is decreasing, the death rate for all cancers combined continue to be 33% higher in African American men and 16% higher in African American women than in white men and women, respectively.[22]

Racial differences in overall cancer death rates are largely seen in breast and colorectal cancers in women and prostate, lung, bronchial, and colorectal cancers in men. Recently, death rates for lung and prostate cancers have decreased faster in African American men than in white men. These decreases have contributed to the recent narrowing of the disparity in cancer mortality between African American and white men. However, in contrast to lung and prostate cancers, the gap has widened for colorectal cancer in both men and women and for breast cancer in women. African American women were 10% less likely to have been diagnosed with breast cancer; however, they were 34% more likely to die of the disease. Breast cancer is the most commonly diagnosed cancer among African American women.[22] This difference accounts for more than one-third (37%) of the overall disparity in cancer mortality between African American and white women.[22] The higher breast cancer mortality rate among African American women occurs despite a lower incidence rate.

Factors that contribute to the higher death rates among African American women include differences in access to and use of early detection and treatment, and differences in tumor characteristics.[44] According to American Cancer Society, the 5-year relative survival rate for breast cancer among African American women is 77%, compared with 90% among whites.[22] Studies have documented unequal receipt of prompt, high-quality treatment for African American women as the major factor in survival rates.[50,51] African Americans are 1.9 times more likely to be diagnosed with diabetes, and 37% of African American men and 41% of African American women are more likely to have hypertension than their white counterparts. Stress is cited as a major contributor to high blood pressure.[7,22,47,50]

Mortality is higher and survival rates are lower in African Americans for most diseases. Although African Americans consist of only 13% of the total United States population, they accounted for 47% of HIV/AIDS cases in 2006. African Americans are twice as likely as their white counterparts to have a stroke and 60% more likely to die of a stroke. African Americans visit the emergency room for asthma-related causes 4.5 times more than whites and are three times as likely to die of an asthmatic attack.[52] Preterm birth and low-birth-weight rates are three times greater for African American women compared with whites.[23] African Americans have a higher incidence of obesity. Although life expectancy has improved greatly for all Americans during the last century, it remains consistently lower for African Americans, at 69.5 years for men and 76.5 years for women.[22,47,52,53]

African Americans have less access to appropriate health care, including preventative care. Therefore, they are not only more susceptible to disease and illness but also more likely to die from them. Even when the incident rate is lower for a disease, such as leukemia, the death rates are higher because of lack of access to appropriate health care.

The difference in drug metabolism rate and treatment are crucial aspects of cultural awareness. Most clinical trials are conducted on white men, and therefore results may not accurately reflect the rate at which African Americans respond to or metabolize drugs. For example, African Americans respond to or metabolize antihypertensives, β-blockers, and psychotropic drugs differently from whites.[54] Studies using drugs metabolized by cytochrome P450 2D6 (CYP2D6) show that many people of African descent metabolize these drugs slower than Caucasians. Therefore, when prescribed the same doses as Caucasians, approximately 40% of people of African descent are predicted to have higher blood levels of drugs metabolized by CYP2D6. Higher blood levels of psychotropic drugs are associated more with side effects, such as sedation, cardiovascular effects, and movement disorders, than with usefulness, increasing the risk associated with these drugs.[54]

Furthermore, African Americans are known to metabolize alcohol differently. Stewart[54] concluded that aspartate aminotransferase and gamma-glutamyltransferase levels elevate more in African Americans after drinking, increasing the risk of death from cirrhosis. Therefore, differences in response to drugs must be considered when treating patients.

CULTURAL SKILL

Cultural skill is the process of learning how to provide culturally appropriate care. It allows for collection of culturally relevant data regarding the patient's health history, thereby enabling nurses to perform a culturally based physical assessment using a culturally sensitive approach. According to Campinha-Bacote,[20] "the goal of a cultural assessment is to determine how the patient defines illness." Assessment is vital to skillfully implementing culturally competent care. Nurses should be cognizant of how skin color variations influence collection of appropriate data. Nurses are trained to perform physical assessments to help diagnose problems; however, most of the skills are based on assessing European skin, and therefore nurses may have a lack of sensitivity and specificity when assessing patients with darkly pigmented skin. African Americans include more than 100 racial strains, lending to skin variations from very dark to very light.[20,25] Assessing African American skin requires diverse skills, such as palpating the skin for warmth and tightness when evaluating for inflammation instead of looking for red discoloration,[39] and examining the oral mucosa or conjunctiva when monitoring for cyanosis instead of noting skin color changes. When observing for jaundice in African Americans, nurses should check the sclera and soles of feet for yellowish discoloration, and pallor is more accurately determined by a lack of reddish tone, which yields ashen to yellowish brown color.[20,25,39] In a study on decubitus ulcers, Ayello[55] found inadequate attention was placed on stage 1 pressure ulcers in persons with darkly pigmented skin. This is because clinicians erroneously believed that dark skin tolerates pressure better than lighter skin. Consequently, those with darker pigmentation had an increased severity and incidence of higher-stage pressure ulcers.[55] Furthermore, dark-skinned patients may have freckles or pigmented streaks in nails, and their nails tend to be thicker; these attributes might be misinterpreted by nurses as abnormal and lead to a misdiagnosis.

Physical assessments should be completed in a culturally sensitive manner. Nurses usually interact with patients using a linear, sequential, and compartmentalized thought process. Questions such as "Tell me what happened first, then next" are asked, and the answers usually require personal information. African Americans view this pattern of sequential and unidirectional information as sequential data gathering, uncaring, and offensive, potentially interfering with obtaining appropriate information during a physical examination. Nonverbal communication, such as eye movement, facial gestures, hand and body language, are used extensively by African Americans. Frequently this nonverbal communication can be overpowering to nurses and lead to a misunderstanding.[39,56] Therefore, when performing an assessment, nurses must be culturally sensitive in their manner and skills.

CULTURAL ENCOUNTERS

Cultural encounters promote "doing" and being involved. They encourage purposeful cultural interactions. Campinha-Bacote[20,37] further asserts that all encounters are cultural when they allow existing knowledge to be validated, refined, and modified to reduce and or prevent stereotyping.

Achieving effective encounters with patients from ethnically and culturally diverse backgrounds is a core component of cultural competence in the clinical setting. According to Campinha-Bacote,[20] "face-to-face interactions that allow for mindful intercultural communications" are necessary. Factors such as language, cultural norms, and concepts of personal space are important variables to consider when encountering African American patients. Facial expressions vary greatly between cultures. African Americans tend to use a smile or other facial gestures to convey feelings. Use of eyes, hands, and body movements are common and may be misinterpreted and can negatively impact the nurse–patient relationship. Furthermore, nurses should not misinterpret high volume of voices as anger, when in fact, this reflects the dramatic manner of expression.

Nurses must understand that African Americans consider being addressed on a first name basis by a stranger, such as the nurse, inappropriate and disrespectful. African Americans, and especially those who are older, prefer to be called by their surname, family name, or professional name until they give permission to do otherwise.[14,27] Being referred to by their family name is a source of pride; being asked how they prefer to be addressed conveys respect.

When African Americans encounter negative experiences, such as miscommunication with nurses, it can influence their health care decisions. Although problems associated with cultural variations in verbal and nonverbal communication styles have been well documented, nurses tend to relate to all clients from an ethnocentric perspective. Differences in communication such as language, dialect, grammatical structure, and pronunciations can negatively impact the encounter between nurse and patient.[27] Although the dominant language spoken by African Americans is English, many studies have shown a bias, unconscious or conscious, exists against African American dialect, especially for those who speak "Black English or Ebonics," which is believed to be inferior to Standard American English.[20] As a result, many African Americans are misunderstood, misinterpreted, and often viewed as uneducated. Conflicts in communication may hinder the nurse–patient/family relationship, and prevent effective cultural encounters.

Patterns of interaction can also interfere with communication. Appropriateness of touch is influenced by culture. In traditional African American culture, touch is extremely important; it conveys approval, caring, trust, and respect. Nurses should observe the response of individuals to determine the appropriateness of touch.[27,39]

The concept of space is greatly influenced by culture, encompassing the individual, body, and surroundings. Ethnic groups differ in their need for space. For example, African Americans are relational and tactile-oriented. Touch and sitting or standing close to another is reported to be acceptable. These behaviors are also related to locus of control. Families often make health-related decisions instead of the patients.[39] This dynamic can present a problem for nurses, who expect patients to be the decision-makers about health-related issues. In the African American culture, extended family and sometimes clergy are involved in health-related decisions.

During encounters, nurses should consider that time is viewed as circular rather than linear. Being present is more important than being on time, which can present problems when scheduling follow-up appointments. Time also relates to patterns.

Nurses tend to function in a monochromic pattern, in which the focus is linear, task-oriented, and sequential; prioritizing one task at a time. However, African Americans tend to follow a polychromic pattern of time, in which the focus is on relationships and connection, rather than tasks.[14,27] African Americans tend to be more present- than future-oriented.

Health literacy is important to consider when encountering African Americans in the health care system. Literature supports a correlation between health literacy and health status. According to the U.S. Department of Health & Human Services, health literacy is defined as the degree to which individuals have the capacity to obtain, process, and understand basic health information needed to make appropriate health decisions and services needed to prevent or treat illness.[26] Patients with low health literacy may have difficulty locating providers and services, filling out complex health forms, sharing their medical history with providers, understanding directions on medicine, knowing the connection between high-risk behaviors and health, and seeking preventive health care. Thus, poor health literacy is considered a key obstruction to receiving optimal health care for African Americans.

SUMMARY
Accepting the Challenge

If nurses show understanding and respect for cultural beliefs, behaviors and practices, even without sanctioning them, this can help promote respect and trust in clinical practice with African Americans. Uncertainty about seeking health care can be reduced through creating trusting relationships between nurses and patients, grounded in nurses' understanding of particular aspects of the African American culture.

The challenge of achieving culturally competent care in a multicultural society requires several different skill sets. Specific knowledge of African American communities, culture, and history is crucial to achieving culturally competent care. The unique and complex relationship that belief systems, especially religious ones, have a to health care must be considered for all patients, but especially African Americans. However, the African American population is not homogenous. Although historically the concept of race was erroneously thought to reflect biologic differences, it is also understood to be a social construct. Therefore, when discussing African Americans or any ethnic group, one must avoid stereotyping and recognize the existence of subcultures within any ethnic group.

Although becoming culturally competent is a complex journey, it offers tremendous rewards. This journey starts with learning about self in an engaging and candid way and gaining knowledge about the cultures of the people being served. Cultural competence is not achieved through words alone, but also through knowledge and the application of that knowledge through cultural encounters. Cultural competence allows cultural information to be obtained in a culturally competent manner, and that knowledge to be used to improve quality of care and health outcomes.

A vital ingredient in cultural competence is experience. Cultural competence cannot be achieved simply through gaining knowledge; encounters must occur. The best teacher is firsthand experience with a culture, if not immersion in it.[34–38] As with many other lessons, one must touch it, try it, and internalize what was learned, and then try again. Nurses must remember that cultural competence is a journey, not a destination; a process, not an event; and a process of *becoming* competent, not *being* culturally competent.[20] Nurses must want to become culturally competent to truly do so. It is reasonable to expect that culturally competent health care will reduce disparities in health outcomes and promote an overall healthier population.

REFERENCES

1. Cook C. The many faces of diversity: overview and summary. Online J Issues Nurs 2003;81(1):1.
2. Culture, Language and Health Literacy. U.S. Department of Health and Human Services Web site. Available at: www.hrsa.gov/culturalcompetence. Accessed February 1, 2011
3. Pacquiao D. The relationship between cultural competence education and increasing diversity in nursing schools and practice settings. J Transcult Nurs 2007;18(1):288–375.
4. Lowe J. Cultural diversity: the intention of nursing. Nurs Forum 2009;44(1):11–8.
5. Culturally Competent Nursing Care: A Cornerstone of Caring. U.S. Department of Health & Human Services Web site. Available at: https://ccnm.thinkculturalhealth.hhs.gov/. Accessed March, 2011.
6. usgovernment spending.com. Available at: http://www.usgovernmentspending.com/. Accessed December 2010. p. 1.
7. National Center for Health Disparities. Eliminating Health Disparities. Evaluating the Economic causes and consequences of Racial and Ethnic heath disparities. American Public Health Association (APHA); 2008. Available at: http://www.apha.org/advocacy/priorities/issues/disparities/. Accessed March, 2011.
8. Paniagua C, Taylor R. Online J Issues Nurs 2008;13(1). 2(51).
9. American Academy of Nursing Expert Panel on Culturally Competent Nursing Care. Culturally competent healthcare. Nurs Outlook 1992;40(6):227–83.
10. Public policy agenda 2009–2010. National League for Nursing (NLN) Web site. Available at: http://www.nln.org/governmentaffairs/pdf/public_policy.pdf. p. 3.
11. US Department of Health & Human Services. National Partnership to end health disparities. Available at: http://minorityhealth.hhs.gov/npa/templates/browse.aspx?lvl=1&lvlid=13. Accessed March 3, 2011.
12. African American Population. BlackDemographics.com. Available at: http://blackdemographics.com/. Accessed November 2010.
13. Population Profile of the United States. U.S. Census Bureau Web site. Available at: http://www.census.gov/population/www/pop-profile/natproj.html. Accessed December, 2010.
14. Wilson L. Cultural diversity: teaching students to provide culturally competent nursing care. In: Caputi L, editor. Teaching nursing: the art and science. 2nd edition. College of DuPage Press; 2008.
15. American Nurses Association. Competencies for health professionals: a multicultural perspective in the promotion of breast, cervical, colorectal and skin health. Washington, DC: ANA Document; 1996.
16. US Census Bureau. National sample survey of registered nurses. Washington, DC: Government Printing Office. Available at: http://bhpr.hrsa.gov/healthworkforce/rnsurvey/2008/. Accessed February 1, 2011.
17. Eisner A, Ellis G. Viewpoint: cultural competence and the African American experience with health care: the case for specific content in cross-cultural education. Acad Med 2007;82(2):176–83.
18. Health resources and services administration. U.S. Department of Health & Human Services Web site. Available at: http://www.aacn.nche.edu/media/FactSheets/NursingShortage.htm. Accessed November, 2010.

19. U.S. Department of Health & Human Services. Bureau of Health Professionals Division of Nursing. National Sample of Registered Nursing; 2010.
20. Campinha-Bacote JA. Culturally competent model of care for African Americans. Urology Nursing 2009;29(1):49–54.
21. Stacks J, Salgado M, Holmes S. Cultural competence and social justice. A partnership for change. Transitions 2004;15(3):4–5.
22. Cancer Facts & Figures for African Americans. American Cancer Society Web site. Available at: http://www.cancer.org/Research/CancerFactsFigures/CancerFactsFigures/cancer-facts-and-figures. Accessed November, 2010.
23. Ngui E, Cortright A, Blair K. An investigation of paternity status and other factors associated with racial and ethnic disparities in birth outcomes in Milwaukee, Wisconsin. Matern Child Health J 2009;13(4):467–78.
24. Andrew M, Boyle J. Transcultural concepts in nursing care. 5th edition. Philadelphia: Wolters Kluwer/Lippincott. Williams & Wilkins; 2008.
25. Purnell L, Paulanka B. Transcultural healthcare: a culturally competent approach. 2nd edition. Philadelphia: F.A. Davis; 2003.
26. Healthy People 2020: The Road Ahead. U.S. Department of Health & Human Services Web site. Available at: http://www.healthypeople.gov/hp2020/. Accessed November, 2010.
27. Giger J, Davidhizar R. Transcultural nursing: assessment and interventions. 5th edition. St. Louis (MO): Moby; 2004.
28. Thomas SB, Quinn SC. The Tuskegee Syphilis Study 1932–1972, implications for HIV education in the black community. Am J Public Health 1991;81:1498–505.
29. Gamble VN. Under the shadow of Tuskegee: African Americans and health care. Am J Public Health 1997;87:1773–8.
30. Kavanagh K. Neither here nor there. The story of a health professional's experience with getting care and needing care. In: Diekelmann NL, editor. First do no harm, Power, oppression, and violence in healthcare. Madison (WI): University of Wisconsin Press; 2002. p. 49–117.
31. Watts R. Race consciousness and the health of African Americans. Online J Issues Nurs 2003;8(1):4.
32. Byrd W, Clayton L. An American health dilemma: a medical history of African Americans and the problem of race: beginnings to 1990. New York: Rutledge; 2000.
33. Leininger M. Transcultural nursing: concepts, theories, research, practice. 2nd edition. New York: McGraw-Hill; 1995.
34. Leininger M, McFarland M. Transcultural nursing: concepts, theories, research and practice. 3rd edition. New York: McGraw-Hill Medical Publishing Division; 2002.
35. Leininger M. Transcultural nursing: the study and practice field. Imprint 1991; 38(2):55–66.
36. Campinha-Bacote J. The process of cultural competence in the delivery of healthcare services. 4th edition. Cincinnati (OH): Transcultural C.A.R.E. Associates; 1998.
37. Campinha-Bacote J. The process of cultural competence in the delivery of healthcare services: a model of care. J Transcult Nurs 2002;13:181–4.
38. Campinha-Bacote J. A culturally conscious approach to holistic nursing. Presented at the American Holistic Nurses Association 2005 Conference June 16–19, 2005. King of Prussia, Pennsylvania.
39. Geiger J, Davidhizar R. Transcultural nursing: assessment in intervention. St. Louis (MO): Mosby-Year Book; 1991.

40. Smedley B, Stith A, Nelson A. Unequal treatment: confronting racial and ethical disparities in healthcare. Washington, DC: National Academy Press; 2002.
41. Koenig HG. Religious attitudes and practices of hospitalized medically ill older adults. Int J Geriatric Psychiatry 1998;13:213–24.
42. George LK, Ellison CG, Larson DB. Explaining the relationships between religious involvement and health. Inquiry 2002;13:190–200.
43. Newlin K, Knafl K, Melkus GD. African American spirituality. ANS Adv Nurs Sci 2000;25:57–70.
44. Lannin DR, Mathews HF, Mitchell J, et al. Influence of socioeconomic and cultural factors in racial differences in late-stage presentation of breast cancer. JAMA 1998;279:1801–7.
45. Kinney AY, Emery G, Dudley WN, et al. Screening behaviors among African-American women at high risk for breast cancer: do beliefs in God matter? Oncol Nurs Forum 2002;29:835–43.
46. Polzer R, Miles MS. Spirituality and self-management of diabetes in African Americans. J Holist Nurs 2005;23(2):230–50 [discussion: 251–4; quiz: 226–7].
47. Cancer Facts & Figures for African Americans 2009–2010. American Cancer Society Web site. Available at: http://www.cancer.org/acs/groups/content/@nho/documents/document/cffaa20092010pdf.pdf. Accessed November 25, 2010.
48. Goldberg J, Hayes W, Huntley J. Understanding health disparities. Health Policy Institute of Ohio; 2004. 4–5.
49. Underwood S, Buseh A, Canales M, et al. Nursing contributions to the elimination of health disparities among African Americans: review and critique of a decade of research. Part III. J Natl Black Nurses Assoc 2005;16(2):35–59.
50. Joslyn SA. Racial differences in treatment and survival from early stage breast cancer. Cancer 2002;95(8):1759–66.
51. Lund MJ, Brawley OP, Ward KC, et al. Parity and disparity in first course treatment of invasive breast cancer. Breast Cancer Res Treat 2008;109(3):545–57.
52. Asthma and Allergy Foundation of America and the National Pharmaceutical Council. Ethnic disparities in the burden and treatment of asthma. Washington, DC; 2006.
53. Bradford LD. Race, genetics, metabolism: drug therapy and clinical trials. MIWatch Web site. Available at: http://www.miwatch.org/2008/04/race_genetics_metabolism_drug_1.html. Accessed November, 2010.
54. Stewart S. Racial and ethical differences in alcohol-associated aspartate aminotransferase and gamma-glutamyltransferase elevation. Arch Intern Med 2002;162(19):2236–9.
55. Ayello E. Predicting pressure ulcer risk. Hartford Institution for Geriatric Nursing Web site 2007;(5). Available at: http://consultgerirn.org/uploads/File/trythis/try_this_5.pdf. Accessed February 1, 2011.
56. Shumate P. Cultural and Diversity: unique challenges in critical care education. Crit Care Nurs Clin North Am 2001;13(1):63–72.

Using Structural Equation Modeling to Identify Predictors of Sexual Behaviors Among Hispanic Men Who Have Sex with Men

Joseph P. De Santis, PhD, ARNP, ACRN*, Adriana Arcia, BSN, RN,
Amber Vermeesch, MSN, RN, NP-C, Karina A. Gattamorta, PhD

KEYWORDS

• Hispanics • Sexual behaviors • Structural Equation Modeling

---

Men who have sex with men (MSM) are at an increased risk of contracting HIV infection and other sexually transmitted infections (STIs) because of participation in high-risk sexual behaviors.[1] High-risk sexual behaviors include sexual activity without condoms, anal intercourse, or sexual behaviors under the influence of drugs and alcohol.[1] Participation in high-risk sexual behaviors places MSM of all ages, races, and ethnicities at risk for HIV and STIs, but Hispanic MSM are at a particular risk of HIV infection related to a number of factors including behavioral, cultural, social, and socioeconomic factors affecting Hispanic MSM.[2] The rate of new cases of HIV infection among Hispanic MSM (27.7/100,000) was nearly triple the rate of new cases of HIV infection among White MSM (9.2/100,000); nearly 60% of all new infections of HIV are among Hispanic MSM.[2]

A number of research studies have been conducted on the sexual behaviors of the general population of MSM, but less is known about the predictors of sexual behaviors among Hispanic MSM. Drawing on the available research knowledge base of the general population of MSM and research with Hispanic MSM when available, a review

---

Funding acknowledgment: This study was funded by the University of Miami General Research Support Award (GRSA). Joseph De Santis, PI. Support for this research was received from the Center of Excellence for Health Disparities Research: EL CENTRO, National Center on Minority Health and Health Disparities Grant P60MD002266.
The authors have nothing to disclose.
University of Miami School of Nursing and Health Studies, 5030 Brunson Drive, Coral Gables, FL 33146, USA
* Corresponding author.
E-mail address: jdesantis@miami.edu

of the literature was conducted before study development to identify variables to include in this study.

REVIEW OF THE LITERATURE
Alcohol Abuse and Sexual Behaviors

In the general population of MSM, alcohol use and abuse have been associated with participation in unprotected anal intercourse (UAI), a high-risk sexual behavior. In a national survey of MSM (n = 2916), a large number of the participants reported alcohol usage before and during sexual behaviors (49%; n = 1412). Those participants who reported alcohol use and abuse were more likely to engage in UAI (odds ratio [OR] = 1.9, 95% confidence interval [CI] = 1.7–2.3).[3]

Only one study that examined the influence of drugs and alcohol on the sexual behaviors of Hispanic MSM could be located. In a study of 193 Hispanic MSM, those who used drugs and alcohol were more likely to participate in high-risk sexual behaviors (OR = 1.8, 95% CI = 1.31–2.49).[4]

Body Image and Sexual Behaviors

In a study conducted with the general population of MSM (n = 535), those MSM who reported an average body image were more likely to engage in UAI than those men who reported an obese body image (13.3% vs 21.6%; $P<.01$).[5] In another study of a sample of the general population of MSM (n = 316), researchers reported that normal weight or overweight men were more likely to engage in UAI than obese men (OR = 3.6, 95% CI = 1.08–12.20). Using bivariate regression analysis, the researchers concluded that men with a higher or more positive body image were more likely to engage in UAI than those with a lower or negative body image (OR = 1.4).[6] Studies that examined the influence of body image, body mass index, or exercise on the sexual behaviors of Hispanic MSM are lacking.

Depression, Self-esteem, and Sexual Behaviors

In a study conducted with a predominantly Hispanic sample of MSM (n = 155), depressive symptoms and self-esteem influenced sexual behaviors. Depressive symptoms accounted for 14.4% of the variance in sexual behaviors ($R^2 = 0.144$, F [1, 203] = 4.312, $P = .039$) and self-esteem accounted for 17% of the variance in sexual behaviors ($R^2 = .170$, F[1, 203] = 6.076, $P = .015$).[7]

Eating Attitudes/Behaviors and Sexual Behaviors

Studies that have examined the relationship of eating attitudes/behaviors and sexual behaviors are nonexistent. MSM have a higher risk for eating disorders than heterosexual men,[8,9] but little is known about eating attitudes/behaviors among Hispanic MSM as well as the influence of eating attitudes/behaviors on sexual behaviors in this subpopulation of MSM.

HIV Status and Sexual Behaviors

Two recent studies that examined the influence of HIV status on the sexual behaviors of Hispanic MSM were identified. Carballo-Dieguez and colleagues[10] compared HIV-infected (n = 50) and HIV-uninfected Hispanic MSM (n = 200) in terms of sexual negotiation and condom usage. The HIV-infected men had significantly more sexual partners than men without HIV infection (M = 6.1 vs 1.5, $t[35]$ = –2.07, P = .046). HIV-infected men were more likely to request that partners refrain from condom usage (χ^2 [1, N = 115] = 4.40, P = .035).

Another study explored the impact of HIV medications, HIV viral load, and sexual risk practices of 395 Hispanic MSM. HIV-infected men were twice as likely to report insertive unprotected anal intercourse than men who were not infected with HIV or men who were not aware of their HIV status (OR = 2.04, 95% CI 1.07–3.87). No relationship was found between receptive anal intercourse and HIV status.[11]

Demographic Variables and Sexual Behaviors

Evidence of the influence of certain demographic variables on sexual behaviors among the general population of MSM can be found in the literature. Kelly and colleagues[12] reported that MSM who were younger in age and had lower levels of education were more likely to participate in high-risk sexual behaviors. In the general population of MSM, income did not have any influence on sexual behaviors.[13]

When conducting research with Hispanic populations, it is important to consider the influence of acculturation as a demographic variable. Instruments have been developed to measure levels of acculturation among Hispanics, but proxy measures of acculturation such as length of time in the United States and language preference and fluency can be used to assess acculturation.[14] Among Hispanic MSM, the combined influence of a preference for Spanish language and foreign birth accounted for 2.3% of the variance in sexual behaviors ($R^2 = 0.023$, $F[2, 200] = 3.420$, $P = .035$).[7] Limited English proficiency[15] and recent immigration[16] have been associated with high-risk sexual behaviors. Length of time living in the United States and language preference were collected as proxy measures of acculturation for this study.

This study was designed to test a conceptual model (**Fig. 1**) that predicts the sexual behaviors of Hispanic MSM. This conceptual model is rooted in the epidemiologic theory of the Web of Causation.[17,18] The Web of Causation, which is based on systems theory, states that single explanations of health conditions or health-risk conditions are not adequate to explain how and why these conditions occur. Instead, there is an interrelatedness of physical, psychological, and social factors, causes, and contributing factors to health and health-risk conditions. The goal of this theory is to find the interrelated causes of health conditions and health risks that may be altered through an intervention to decrease the sequel of these health conditions.

METHOD
Sample

A convenience sample of 100 community-dwelling Hispanic MSM ages 18 and older ($M = 32.47$, SD $\pm$ 7.29, range = 18–51) who resided in South Florida participated in the study. A more complete demographic profile of the study's participants is included in **Table 1**.

Measures

Six instruments and the demographic questionnaire were used in this study. The instruments were chosen to operationalize the study variables of alcohol abuse, body image, depression, eating attitudes and behaviors, self-esteem, and sexual behaviors. Alcohol abuse was measured by the CAGE Questionnaire.[19] Body image was assessed by the Adonis Complex Questionnaire (ACQ).[20] Depressive symptoms were measured by the Center for Epidemiologic Studies-Depressed Mood Scale (CES-D).[21] Eating attitudes and behaviors used to assess risk for eating disorders were measured by the Eating Attitudes Test (EAT-26).[22] Self-esteem was measured using the Rosenberg[23] Self-Esteem Scale (RSES). Sexual behaviors were measured using the Safer Sex Behavior Questionnaire (SSBQ).[24]

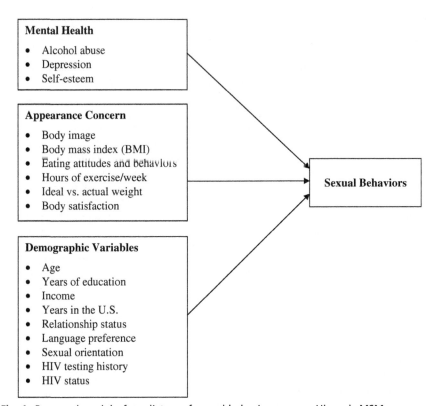

Fig. 1. Proposed model of predictors of sexual behaviors among Hispanic MSM.

The demographic questionnaire included items about age, number of years of education, country of birth, length of time in the United States if foreign-born, income, language preference, sexual orientation, and relationship status. Participants were also asked to report their HIV testing history, HIV status, the number of hours of exercise per week, and height and weight, which were used to calculate body mass index (BMI).[25]

These 6 instruments and the demographic questionnaire were translated into Spanish using a professional translation service as required by the University's Institutional Review Board, and then back-translated into English. Comparison of the back-translated survey to the original English versions is an appropriate method of ensuring accurate translation.[26]

CAGE Questionnaire

The CAGE Questionnaire was used to measure alcohol abuse. This instrument asks participants to respond "yes" or "no" to each of the 4 items. Each "yes" response is scored as 1. Total scores on the CAGE Questionnaire range from 0 to 4. A score of 2 or higher is considered clinically significant for alcohol-related disorders. Sensitivity and specificity of the CAGE Questionnaire range from 0.52 to 0.96 in the general population.[19] For Hispanic populations, reliability coefficients ranging from 0.73 to 0.91 have been reported, and this instrument was 92% sensitive and 74% specific when used with Hispanic populations.[27] The CAGE Questionnaire demonstrated an internal consistency of 0.73 in this sample of Hispanic MSM. The CAGE Questionnaire has been correlated with the Composite International Diagnostic Interview (CIDI) and

Table 1
Demographic characteristics of the sample (n = 100)

Variable	M	SD	Range
Age	32.47	7.29	18–51
Years of education	14.96	2.4	5–20
Income	$40,550.50	$20,932.47	$0–100,000
Years in the United States (if foreign-born)	13.35	9.21	<1–49
Body mass index[a]	25.25	3.44	18.20–37.00
Number of hours of exercise/week	2.68	2.99	0–13
			n and %
Relationship Status			
Single			72
Partnered			28
Birth			
Foreign-born			83
US-born			17
Language Preference			
English			33
Spanish			25
Either English or Spanish			42
Sexual Orientation			
Homosexual			88
Heterosexual			5
Bisexual			7
Tested for HIV During Lifetime			
Yes			92
No			8
Most Recent HIV Test Result			
Negative			84
Positive			6
Unknown			10
Body Satisfaction			
Very dissatisfied			13
Dissatisfied			17
Neutral			20
Satisfied			41
Very satisfied			9
BMI Category[a]			
Underweight			1
Normal weight			44
Overweight			43
Obese			8

[a] n = 96 because of missing data.

biologic markers of alcohol usage such as liver function tests and blood alcohol levels as tests of construct validity.[27]

Adonis Complex Questionnaire

The Adonis Complex Questionnaire (ACQ)[20] was used to measure concerns about body image. This 13-item Likert scale contains scores of 0 (*rarely or not at all*) to 3 (*frequently*). The total scores on the ACQ range from 0 to 39. Higher scores on the ACQ indicate greater concerns with body image. Reliability measures have not been published for the ACQ, but this is the only instrument currently available to measure body image concerns among MSM.[20] The ACQ demonstrated an internal consistency of 0.80 in this sample of Hispanic MSM.

Center for Epidemiologic Studies-Depressed Mood Scale

The Center for Epidemiologic Studies-Depressed Mood Scale (CES-D)[21] was used to measure depressive symptoms. Designed for research purposes, this 20-item Likert scale contains scores from 0 (*rarely or none of the time or <1 day*) to 3 (*most or all of the time or 5 to 7 days*). Total scores on the CES-D range from 0 to 60. CES-D scores greater than 16 indicate higher levels of depressive symptoms. A reliability coefficient of 0.85 for internal consistency has been reported for the general population.[21] With various Hispanic subgroups, reliability coefficients ranging from 0.78 to 0.99 have been reported.[28] In the Hispanic MSM population, a reliability coefficient of 0.88 has been reported.[7] The reliability coefficient of 0.85 was noted in this sample of Hispanic MSM. Validity of the CES-D has been established by correlating the CES-D with other depression and mood scales.[21]

Eating Attitudes Test-26

The Eating Attitudes Test-26 (EAT-26)[22] was used to measure eating attitudes and behaviors and to assess risk for eating disorders. This 26-item Likert scale contains scores from 0 (*sometimes, rarely, or never*) to 3 (*always*). Total scores on the EAT-26 can range from 0 to 78. EAT-26 scores above 20 indicate a high risk for eating disorders. A reliability coefficient of 0.98 for internal consistency has been reported A reliability coefficient of 0.91 was reported with Hispanic women.[29] The EAT-26 demonstrated an internal consistency of 0.93 in this sample of Hispanic MSM. Validity of the EAT-26 has been established by correlating the instrument's subscales with bulimia, weight, body image, and psychological symptoms.[22]

Rosenberg Self-Esteem Scale

The Rosenberg Self-Esteem Scale (RSES)[23] was used to measure self-esteem. This 10-item Likert scale contains scores that range from 0 (*agree*) to 3 (*strongly agree*). The total scores on the RSES range from 0 to 30. Higher scores on the RSES indicate higher levels of self-esteem, and scores less than or equal to 16 indicate lower self-esteem. Reliability coefficients for internal consistency ranging from 0.77 to 0.88 have been reported in the general population, and 0.84 with Hispanic individuals.[30] A reliability coefficient of 0.73 was reported previously with Hispanic MSM.[7] The RSES had an internal consistency of 0.83 in this sample of Hispanic MSM. Validity of the RSES has been established by correlating the RSES with measures of depression, anxiety, and peer relationships.[23]

Safer Sex Behavior Questionnaire

The Safer Sex Behavior Questionnaire (SSBQ)[24] was used to measure sexual behaviors, including condom usage, high-risk sexual behaviors, and sexual communication and negotiation. This 27-items on this Likert scale are each rated on a 4-point scale ranging from 1 (*never*) to 4 (*always*). Total scores on the SSBQ range from 27 to 108. The mean score for men on the SSBQ is 69. Higher scores on the SSBQ indicate participation in safer sex behaviors. A reliability coefficient for internal consistency of 0.82 was reported for a sample of college-age men and women. The SSBQ has not been used with the general Hispanic population, but a reliability coefficient of 0.85

and a mean of 78 has been reported in previous research with Hispanic MSM.[7] The SSBQ had an internal consistency of 0.83 in this sample of Hispanic MSM. Validity of the SSBQ has been established by correlating the SSBQ with measures of self-expression, assertiveness, and risk-taking.[24]

PROCEDURE

Participants were recruited from bars, clubs, and beaches and were invited to participate if they met the inclusion criteria: (1) age 18 years or older; (2) self-identified as Hispanic; (3) able to speak and read either English of Spanish; and (4) reported sexual activity with another man at least once during the lifetime, regardless of sexual orientation.

Once participants met inclusion criteria and received a detailed explanation of the study in their preferred language and agreed to participate by signing an informed consent form, they were given the option to complete the study on-site or to travel to the university for increased privacy. For those who opted to complete the study on-site, privacy was enhanced through the use of clipboards and cover sheets. Seventy-one percent of the participants completed the survey in English, and 29% in Spanish. Participants were compensated $10 at completion of the study.

Surveys were checked for completeness before data analysis began. Complete data were noted for all study variables except body mass index (BMI), which was 96% complete. Mean and mode substitution were used to manage missing demographic data.

DATA ANALYSIS

Data were analyzed to test and modify the measurement model, and test and modify the structural model. Descriptive statistics were generated using the Statistical Package for the Social Sciences (SPSS, Version 18.0, Chicago, IL, USA).

Structural equation modeling (SEM) is based on examining the variance-covariance structure among the observed variables and generating a chi-square test of model fit, an evaluation of the null hypothesis that the covariance matrix in the population is equal to that implied by the model. SEM consists of both measurement equations that relate the observed variables to the latent factors, and latent variable equations that estimate the specified relationships among the latent variables. A number of fit indices are available for assessing structural equation models. One such fit index is the model chi-square. Failure to reject the null hypothesis (ie, $P > .05$) supports the researcher's model. There are limitations with relying solely on the chi-square statistic and as a result, other fit indices have been used to examine the approximate fit of models. The Comparative Fit Index (CFI) is an incremental fit index that measures improvement in model fit of the hypothesized model relative to a baseline model.[31] The CFI has a 0 to 1 range. The standardized root mean square residual (SRMR) and the root mean square error of approximation (RMSEA) are residual-based fit indices that assess how well a model reproduces the sample data by comparing it with a saturated model that exactly reproduces the sample covariance matrix. Hu and Bentler[32] recommended using SRMR in combination with one of the other fit indices to evaluate model fit, along with using the cutoff of CFI greater than 0.95, SRMR less than 0.08, and RMSEA less than 0.06.

Mplus statistical software version 5.21[33] (Los Angeles, CA, USA) was used for subsequent analyses, including the default setting of full information maximum likelihood (FIML) for the handling of missing data of the study variables. A measurement model of 2 latent variables, mental health and appearance concern, was tested before incorporation of the measurement portion into a structural model for which the outcome variable was the total SSBQ score, a measure of sexual behaviors.

RESULTS
Demographic Variables

A complete description of the study's participants is provided in **Table 1**. Participants were asked to self-report actual body weight and to provide their ideal body weight. The mean actual weight for the sample was 80.20 kg (SD $\pm$ 15.86), whereas the reported mean ideal weight was 76.32 kg (SD $\pm$ 14.87). The difference between the actual weight and ideal weight was statistically significant ($t = 3.98$, $df = 91$, $P = .000$).

Study Variables

Total scores on each of the measures of alcohol abuse, eating attitudes and behaviors, body image, depression, self-esteem, and sexual behaviors are illustrated with descriptive statistics. Results are presented in **Table 2**. A variance-covariance matrix of the study variables is shown in **Table 3**.

Using the criteria established for each of the measures of alcohol abuse, body image, depression, eating attitudes and behaviors, and self-esteem, a number of the participants were at risk for these health conditions. The results indicated that 18% were at risk for alcohol abuse; 29% had body image concerns; 25% had high levels of depressive symptoms; 13% of the study participants were at risk for an eating disorder; and 12% reported low levels of self-esteem.

The measure of sexual behaviors (the SSBQ) does not have "cut-off" values to determine low versus high levels of safer sex behaviors. The original study reported means for males of 68.0 to 69.2. Standard deviations were not reported.[24] A study with a sample of Hispanic MSM (n = 155) that used the SSBQ reported a mean of 79.3 (SD $\pm$ 12.6, range = 46–104).[34] This study's mean 75.14 (SD $\pm$ 11.96, range = 48–103) is slightly lower, indicating that the men in this current study are engaging in slightly lower levels of safer sex behavior compared with the sample studied by De Santis and colleagues.[34]

Measurement Model Testing

The first step in structural equation modeling is testing the measurement model. If the measurement model does not fit the data, structural modeling testing cannot be performed.

Table 2
Alcohol abuse, body image, depression, eating attitudes and behaviors, self-esteem, and sexual behaviors of the sample (n = 100)

Variable	Measure	Scale Range	Percent
Alcohol abuse	CAGE	0–2	90
		3–4	10

Variable	Measure	Scale Range	Mean (SD)
Body image	ACQ	0–39	7.11 ($\pm$ 5.94)
Depression	CES-D	0–31	12.23 ($\pm$ 8.35)
Eating attitudes and behaviors	EAT-26	0–75	11.20 ($\pm$ 13.66)
Self-esteem	RSE	8–30	22.81 ($\pm$ 5.58)
Sexual behaviors	SSBQ	48–103	75.14 ($\pm$ 11.96)

Abbreviations: ACQ, Adonis Complex Questionnaire; CES-D, Center for Epidemiologic Studies Depressed Mood Scale; EAT, Eating Attitudes Test; RSES, Rosenberg Self-Esteem Scale; SSBQ, Safer Sex Behavior Questionnaire.

Table 3
Variance-covariance matrix of the study variables

	RSES	CES-D	CAGE	EAT-26	ACQ	BMI	SSBQ
RSES	30.874	—	—	—	—	—	—
CES-D	−32.774	74.148	—	—	—	—	—
CAGE	−0.717	2.742	1.167	—	—	—	—
EAT-26	−27.768	35.023	5.557	186.362	—	—	—
ACQ	−4.949	10.892	1.269	32.535	34.958	—	—
BMI	4.300	-8.061	−0.859	−9.456	−3.791	11.825	—
SSBQ	26.017	−35.589	−3.011	−41.883	−8.835	4.952	141.540

Abbreviations: ACQ, Adonis Complex Questionnaire; BMI, Body Mass Index; CES-D, Center for Epidemiologic Studies Depressed Mood Scale; EAT, Eating Attitudes Test; RSES, Rosenberg Self-Esteem Scale; SSBQ, Safer Sex Behavior Questionnaire.

Total scores from the CES-D, a measure of depression, and total RSES scores, a measure of self-esteem, were specified as indicators of a latent variable labeled mental health. Positive mental health was defined by high self-esteem scores and low depression scores. Mental health had a strong negative correlation ($B = -0.533$, $P<.001$) with a latent variable labeled appearance concern. Mental health was associated with higher RSES scores ($B = 0.861$, $P<.001$) and lower CES-D scores ($B = -0.795$, $P<.001$).

The indicators of appearance concern were specified as total EAT-26 scores (eating attitudes and behaviors), total ACQ scores (body image), and BMI scores. High levels of concern over appearance were associated with increased EAT-26 ($B = 0.753$, $P<.001$), ACQ scores ($B = 0.514$, $P<.001$), and decreased BMI ($B = -0.315$, $P<.05$). The metric for both latent variables was set by fixing their respective variances to 1, thereby allowing a loading to be generated for each indicator. The measurement model **(Fig. 2)** had good fit to the data ($\chi^2[4] = 5.120$, $P = .275$; CFI = 0.998; RMSEA = 0.053; SRMR = 0.042).

Eating attitudes and behaviors are at the conceptual crossroads between concern over appearance and mental illness. Therefore, total EAT-26 scores justifiably could have been used as indicators for either appearance concern or mental health. The authors chose to specify total EAT scores as indicators of appearance concern because although the instrument taps aspects of mental health and illness, the content of the items is conceptually closer to appearance concern. Furthermore,

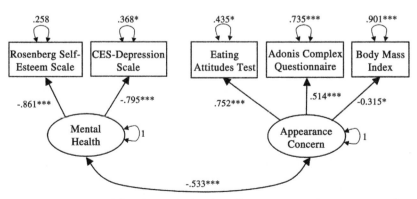

Fig. 2. Measurement model with standardized coefficients. Rectangles represent indicators of latent variables, which are shown in ovals. *$P<.05$. ***$P<.001$.

specifying total EAT-26 scores as indicators of mental health led to a model with significantly poorer fit with the data, based on the result of a chi-square difference test, than the model that was retained.

Several alternative measurement models were attempted and rejected. Total CAGE scores, a measure of alcohol abuse, failed to fit the data as indicators of mental health. Two potential indicators of appearance concern were rejected because of poor model fit: hours of exercise per week and the absolute value of the difference between actual and ideal body weight. A single-item measure of body satisfaction ("How satisfied are you with your body?") achieved model fit as an indicator of appearance concern. However, the loading on the indicator was not significant and it was replaced with BMI, which led to both a significant loading and equally good model fit.

Structural Model Testing

A structural model in which sexual behaviors, as measured by the total SSBQ scores, was predicted by CAGE scores, mental health, and appearance concern fit the data well ($\chi^2[10] = 14.498$, $P = .152$; CFI = 0.966; RMSEA = 0.067; SRMR = 0.043). The model, with standardized coefficients, is shown in **Fig. 3**. Of the 3 possible direct paths to sexual behaviors (mental health, CAGE scores [alcohol abuse], and appearance concern), only the direct path from mental health to sexual behaviors was significant ($B = 0.392$, $P<.01$). Covariances between mental health and CAGE scores ($B = -0.216$, $P = .08$); mental health and appearance concern ($B = -0.530$, $P<.001$); and CAGE scores and appearance concern ($B = .488$, $P<.001$) were also noted. Although the only significant direct path to sexual behaviors was mental health, there is shared variance among the variables of mental health, alcohol abuse, and appearance concern that is not being captured by the measures that were used in this study to define these variables.

Table 4 contains the unstandardized path coefficients, standard errors and z values for the structural model. Because the sample size is somewhat small for this type of analysis, the authors assigned the indicator loadings from the measurement model and specified them as starting values for the structural model. This strategy led to model convergence that did not occur without the specification of starting values.

Owing to the scarcity of literature regarding Hispanic MSM, a partially exploratory approach to model specification was taken. Models were tested in which the respondents' relationship status (partnered or not) and HIV testing history (ever had an HIV test) were specified as predictors of sexual behaviors (total SSBQ scores), but rejected because relationship status and HIV testing history failed to fit the data. Similarly, neither age, education, income, nor number of years in the United States generated good model fit when specified as predictors of sexual behaviors (total SSBQ scores). Furthermore, age was not a good predictor of appearance concern.

DISCUSSION

This study was designed to test a model that could predict the sexual behaviors of Hispanic MSM that was based on the conceptual framework of the Web of Causation.[17,18] It was hypothesized that certain specified factors could predict the sexual behaviors of Hispanic MSM. Measurement and structural models were tested to develop a model that predicts the sexual behaviors of this subpopulation of MSM.

The results of this study support the existing body of research that reports that mental health, expressed in terms of depression and self-esteem, are strong predictors of sexual behaviors among Hispanic MSM.[7] One possible reason that mental health has such a large impact on sexual behaviors of the men in this study may lie in Hispanic culture. In general, Hispanic culture values strong family relationships. Sexual

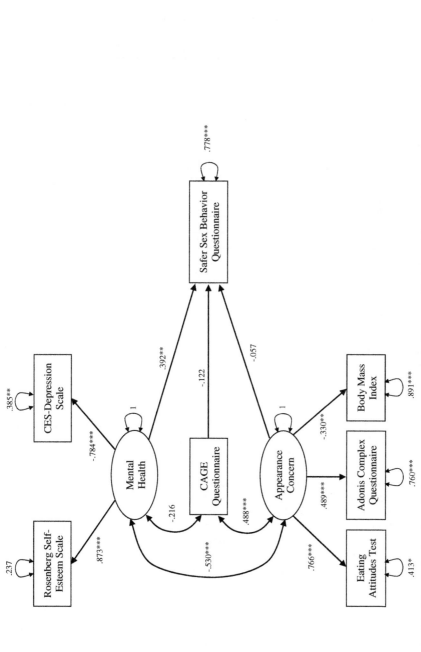

Fig. 3. Structural model with standardized coefficients. Rectangles represent indicators of latent variables, which are shown in ovals. *P<.05. **P<.01. ***P<.001.

Table 4
Unstandardized path coefficients, standard errors and z values for indicator loadings, direct effects, and covariances

	Coefficient	SE	z
Latent variable loadings			
Appearance concern to			
EAT	10.46	1.78	5.89[c]
ACQ	2.89	0.67	4.32[c]
BMI	−1.13	0.44	−2.56[a]
Mental health to			
CES-D	−6.75	0.95	−7.11[c]
RSES	4.85	0.63	7.75[c]
Direct paths			
Mental health to SSBQ	4.66	1.59	2.94[b]
Appearance concern to SSBQ	−0.68	2.01	−0.34
CAGE to SSBQ	−1.34	1.28	−1.05
Covariances			
Mental health with CAGE	−0.23	0.13	−1.77
Mental health with appearance concern	−0.53	0.13	−4.23[c]
CAGE with appearance concern	0.53	0.12	4.58[c]

Abbreviations: ACQ, Adonis Complex Questionnaire; BMI, Body Mass Index; CES-D, Center for Epidemiologic Studies Depressed Mood Scale; EAT, Eating Attitudes Test; RSES, Rosenberg Self-Esteem Scale; SSBQ, Safer Sex Behavior Questionnaire.

[a] $P<.05$.
[b] $P<.01$.
[c] $P<.001$.

orientation may affect these family relationships. Decreased familial support could have an impact on mental health, expressed in terms of depression and self-esteem.[35] Resulting depression and low self-esteem may contribute to high-risk sexual behaviors.[7]

Alcohol abuse was not a direct predictor of sexual behaviors in this sample. Previous research, however, has reported that alcohol use contributed to high-risk sexual behaviors among Hispanic MSM.[4] This was an unexpected finding based on previous research. There are possible explanations for this finding. First, once mental health is controlled, perhaps alcohol abuse is no longer a significant predictor of sexual behaviors. Second, because the participants were recruited in sites where alcohol was readily available, the results regarding alcohol abuse may have been influenced by the study sites, and are not truly representative of alcohol abuse among Hispanic MSM.

A third possible explanation for alcohol abuse not being a predictor of sexual behaviors in this study could be rooted in the measure of sexual behaviors, the SSBQ. The SSBQ contains an item that asks participants if alcohol is used before and during sexual behavior.[24] Variability of the responses within this sample on this particular item on the SSBQ could have captured outcome-specific information, and rendered alcohol abuse, as reflected by the CAGE scores, as insignificant. More research with this population is needed to explore the complex relationship of alcohol use/abuse, mental health, and sexual behaviors of Hispanic MSM.

Body image and eating attitudes and behaviors, other mental health indicators, were not significant predictors of sexual behaviors. However, the latent variable of appearance concern was significantly correlated with mental health. Previous studies to document the influence of appearance concern expressed in body image on the sexual behaviors of Hispanic MSM are lacking, but with the correlation between the latent variables of appearance concern and mental health that was noted in this study, future studies should consider including these correlates of mental health as a cluster. Because the influence of body image or eating attitudes and behaviors on the sexual behaviors of Hispanic MSM has not been previously explored, this study adds some important information to the knowledge base of the health behaviors of these men.

An alternate explanation for the study's findings is that the other predictors that could possibly be used to predict sexual behaviors were not included in this study.[36] The significant correlation between the predictors provides evidence that there is something else within these variables that was not captured by those 3 predictors. Previous research has shown that other factors, such as abuse of substances other than alcohol,[37] childhood sexual abuse,[38] power and control in intimate partner relationships,[39] and a lack of family support[40] have been linked to high-risk sexual behaviors among Hispanic MSM. Because none of these variables were included in this study, further research is needed that tests the influence of these variables on sexual behaviors.

An important strength of this study is that the structural model fit well within the data without regard to demographic variables. Although previous research on Hispanic MSM found that certain demographic variables such as age, education,[12] language preference, foreign birth,[7] limited English proficiency, and recent immigration[16] were related to sexual behaviors among Hispanic MSM, these demographic variables were not significant predictors in this study. Attempts to include these demographic variables (age, income, education, years living in the United States, relationship status, and HIV testing history) all worsened model fit. The parsimony of this model translates into stronger generalizability than a model in which demographic variables were influential on sexual behaviors.

Overall, the results of this study indicate that Hispanic MSM are at risk for a number of physical and psychological health conditions. These include alcohol abuse (18%), body image concerns (29%), depression (25%), risk for eating disorders (13%), and low self-esteem (12%). These results indicate that screening for alcohol abuse, body image disturbance, depression, eating disorders, and low self-esteem in combination with addressing high-risk sexual behaviors is important in providing care to this population. One implication of this study is that health care providers and researchers can use the results to gain a better understanding of the complexity of risk behaviors in this population. Health care providers working with members of this population can use these results as evidence for the need to be aware that clients who are depressed or who report low self-esteem may be at risk for engaging in high-risk sexual behaviors. Researchers can use this model as a starting point from which to explore further the interrelationships of health risk behaviors among Hispanic MSM. Whether through clinical practice or research, more emphasis needs to be placed on reducing participation in high-risk sexual behaviors, which would decrease the rates of HIV infection and other STIs among this population.

NURSING IMPLICATIONS

To provide culturally appropriate care to Hispanic MSM, nurses and other health care providers must appreciate the unique cultural factors that influence high-risk behaviors in this population of MSM. One of the most fundamental factors is familial relationships.[40] To decrease high-risk behaviors, Hispanic MSM need psychosocial support. If this support is not available from the family, nurses should be aware of community-based agencies that can offer services, such as support groups that may serve as a source of psychosocial support.

To cope with the lack of psychosocial support, some Hispanic MSM may use drugs and alcohol.[4] For men with drug and alcohol problems, prompt referrals to mental health providers who can address the use of drugs and alcohol in a culturally sensitive manner is necessary.

In addition to drug and alcohol use, mental health conditions such as altered body image, depression, altered eating attitudes and behaviors, and low self-esteem must be addressed in a culturally appropriate manner. As Hispanic MSM acculturate to US society, the risk for body image disturbance, depression, eating disorders, and low self-esteem increases. Screening for these conditions during health care encounters is necessary. Clients reporting concerns with any of these mental health conditions require prompt referral to mental health professionals who are culturally competent to provide care to this population of men.

Last, nurses and other health care providers must be comfortable assessing for and addressing high-risk sexual behaviors. Some Hispanic MSM may lack basic information about safer sex behaviors, or may not have an accurate perception of risk for HIV and other STIs. As these men acculturate to US society, participation in high-risk sexual behaviors increases.[34] Educating these men in a culturally appropriate manner about HIV/STIs, high-risk versus lower-risk sexual behaviors, and other risk factors may decrease overall risk.

LIMITATIONS

The results of this study provide some important information on predictors of sexual behaviors of Hispanic MSM. Certain limitations of this study are evident. Because the data were collected at one point in time in a cross-sectional design, measurement of change in the variables over time was not possible.[41] The participants were drawn from a convenience sample recruited at selected sites frequented by MSM, so the participants in this study may not be truly representative of the population of Hispanic MSM. The use of convenience sampling is necessary, however, as this sampling method is one of the most effective means of surveying hard-to-reach populations such as Hispanic MSM.[42]

SUMMARY

The results of this study provide some important new information regarding the predictors of sexual behaviors among Hispanic MSM. The final model suggests that mental health is a significant predictor of sexual behaviors in this sample. Major implications for the development of interventions to address high-risk sexual behaviors highlight the need for health care providers and researchers to be cognizant of the influence of mental health issues on sexual behaviors.

ACKNOWLEDGMENTS

The authors thank the following individuals for their assistance in data collection and entry: D. Martin Layerla, BSN, RN; Susana Barroso, BSN, RN; and Michael Sanchez, BSN, RN.

REFERENCES

1. Centers for Disease Control and Prevention. HIV among gay, bisexual and other men who have sex with men (MSM). 2010. Available at: http://www.cdc.gov/hiv/topics/msm/index.htm. Accessed November 24, 2010.

2. Centers for Disease Control and Prevention. HIV/AIDS among Hispanics/Latinos. 2009. Available at: http://www.cdc.gov/hiv/hispanics/index.htm. Accessed November 24, 2010.

3. Hirshfield S, Remein RH, Humberstone M, et al. Substance use and high risk sex among men who have sex with men: a national online study in the USA. AIDS Care 2004;16(8):1036–47.

4. Smolenski DJ, Ross MW, Risser JM, et al. Sexual compulsivity and high risk sex among Latino men who have sex with men: the role of internalized homonegativity and gay organizations. AIDS Care 2009;21(1):42–9.

5. Allensworth-Davis D, Welles SL, Hellerstedt WL, et al. Body image, body satisfaction, and unsafe anal intercourse among men who have sex with men. J Sex Res 2008;45(1):49–56.

6. Kraft C, Robinson BE, Nordstrom DL, et al. Obesity, body image, and unsafe sex in men who have sex with men. Arch Sex Behav 2006;35:587–95.

7. De Santis JP, Colin JM, Vasquez EP, et al. The relationship of depressive symptoms, self-esteem, and sexual behaviors in a predominately Hispanic sample of men who have sex with men. Am J Mens Health 2008;2(4):314–21.

8. Feldman MB, Meyer IH. Eating disorders in diverse lesbian, gay, and bisexual populations. Int J Eat Disord 2007;40(3):218–26.

9. Kaminski PL, Chapman BP, Haynes SD, et al. Body image, eating behaviors, and attitudes toward exercise among gay and straight men. Eat Behav 2005;6(3):179–87.

10. Carballo-Dieguez A, Miner M, Dolezal C, et al. Sexual negotiation, HIV-status disclosure, and sexual risk behavior among Latino men who use the Internet to seek sex with other men. Arch Sex Behav 2006;35(4):473–81.

11. Munoz-Laboy M, Castellanos D, Westacott R. Sexual risk behavior, viral load, and perceptions of HIV transmission among homosexually active Latino men: an exploratory study. AIDS Care 2005;17(1):33–45.

12. Kelly JA, Sikkema KJ, Winett RA, et al. Factors predicting continued high risk sexual behavior among gay men in small cities: psychological, behavioral, and demographic characteristics related to unsafe sex. J Consult Clin Psychol 1995;63(1):101–7.

13. Santelli JS, Lowry R, Brener ND. The association of sexual behaviors of socioeconomic status, family structure, and race/ethnicity among U.S. adolescents. Am J Public Health 2000;90(10):1582–8.

14. Unger JB, Ritt-Olson A, Wagner K, et al. A comparison of acculturation measures among Hispanic/Latino adolescents. J Youth Adolesc 2007;36:555–65.

15. Gullamo-Ramos V, Jaccard J, Pena J, et al. Acculturation-related variables, sexual initiation, and subsequent sexual behavior among Puerto Rican, Mexican, and Cuban youth. Health Psychol 2005;24(1):88–95.

16. Blake SM, Ledsky R, Goodenow C, et al. Recency of immigration, substance use, and sexual behaviors among Massachusetts adolescents. Am J Public Health 2001;91(5):794–8.

17. Engel G. The need for a new medical model: a challenge for biomedicine. Science 1977;196:129–36.

18. Engel G. The clinical application of the biopsychosocial model. Am J Psychiatry 1980;137:535–44.

19. Ewing JA. Detecting alcoholism: the CAGE questionnaire. JAMA 1984;252(14):1905–7.

20. Pope HG, Phillips KA, Olivardia R. The adonis complex: the secret crisis of male body obsession. New York: The Free Press; 2000.

21. Radloff LS. The CES-D scale: a self-report depression scale for research in the general population. Appl Psychol Meas 1977;1(5):385–401.

22. Garner DM, Olmsted MP, Bohr Y, et al. The eating attitudes test: psychometric features and clinical correlates. Psychol Med 1982;12(4):871–88.
23. Rosenberg M. Society and adolescent self-image. Middleton (CT): Wesleyan University Press; 1989.
24. Dilorio C, Parsons M, Lehr S, et al. Measurement of safe sex behavior in adolescents and young adults. Nurs Res 1992;41(4):203–8.
25. Centers for Disease Control and Prevention. Adult BMI calculator: English. 2010. Available at: http://www.cdc.gov/healthyweight/assessing/bmi/adult_bmi/english_bmi_calculator/bmi_calculator.html. Accessed November 24, 2010.
26. Marin G, Marin BV. Research with Hispanic populations. Newbury Park (CA): Sage Publications; 1991.
27. Saitz R, Lepore MF, Sullivan LM, et al. Alcohol abuse and dependence in Latinos living in the United States. Arch Intern Med 1999;159:718–24.
28. Yang FM, Cazola-Lancaster Y, Jones RN. Within-group differences in depression among older Hispanics living in the United States. J Gerontol B Psychol Sci Soc Sci 2008;63(1):P27–32.
29. Joiner GH, Kashubeck S. Acculturation, body image, self-esteem, and eating disorder symptomatology in adolescent Mexican-American women. Psychol Women Q 1996;20(3):419–35.
30. Martin-Albo J, Nunez JL, Navarro JG, et al. The Rosenberg self-esteem scale: translation and validation in university students. Span J Psychol 2007;10(2):458–67.
31. Bollen KA, Curran PJ. Latent curve models: a structural equation approach. New York (NY): Wiley; 1989.
32. Hu L, Bentler PM. Cutoff criteria for fit indexes in covariance structure analysis: conventional criteria versus new alternatives. Struct Equ Modeling 1999;6(1):1–55.
33. Muthen LK, Muthen BO. Mplus user's guide fifth edition. Los Angeles (CA): Muthen & Muthen; 1998-2007.
34. De Santis JP, Vasquez EP, Weidel JJ, et al. A comparison of depressive symptoms, self-esteem, and sexual behaviors between foreign-born and U.S.-born Hispanic men who have sex with men: implications for HIV prevention. Hisp Health Care Int 2009;7(2):80–7.
35. Diaz RM, Ayala G, Bien E, et al. The impact of homophobia, poverty, and racism on the mental health of gay and bisexual Latino men: Findings from three U.S. cities. Am J Public Health 2001;91(6):927–32.
36. Bollen KA. Structural equations with latent variables. New York: John Wiley & Sons; 1989.
37. Akin M, Fernandez MI, Bowen GS, et al. HIV risk behaviors of Latin American and Caribbean men who have sex with men in Miami, Florida. Rev Panam Salud Publica 2008;23:341–8.
38. Dolezal C, Carballo-Dieguez A. Childhood sexual experiences and the perception of abuse among Latino men who have sex with men. J Sex Res 2002;39:165–73.
39. Feldman MB, Diaz RM, Ream GL, et al. Intimate partner violence and HIV behavior among Latino gay and bisexual men. J LGBT Health Res 2007;3(2):9–19.
40. Guarnero PA. Family and community influences on the social and sexual lives of Latino gay men. J Transcult Nurs 2007;18(1):12–8.
41. Creswell JW. Research design: qualitative, quantitative, and mixed methods approaches. 3rd edition. Thousand Oaks (CA): Sage; 2008.
42. De Santis J. Conducting nursing research with men who have sex with men: challenges and strategies for nurse researchers. J Assoc Nurses AIDS Care 2006; 17(6):47–52.

Index

Note: Page numbers of article titles are in **boldface** type.

A

Acculturation, in Hispanic individuals seeking pain management in southwestern border community, **193–199**

Advanced practice nurses, PMN nursing students' knowledge and attitudes on culturally competent care, **201–205**

African Americans, delivering culturally competent care to, **219–232**
    culture and cultural competence, 222–223
    cultural competence theories of care for, 223–229
        cultural awareness, 224
        cultural desire, 224
        cultural encounters, 228–229
        cultural knowledge, 224–227
        cultural skill, 227
    demographic trends and nursing, 220–221
    summary, 229–230
    the African American experience, 221–222

Alcohol abuse, as predictor of sexual behavior in Hispanic men who have sex with men, 36–38

Anthropology, applied or medical, 147–148

Appalachia, views of providers and patients on colorectal cancer screening in rural, **181–192**

Attitudes, of advanced practice psychiatric nursing students on culturally competent care, **201–205**

B

Biomedicine, culture of, 163–164

Border communities, southwestern, acculturation in Hispanic individuals seeking pain management in, **193–199**

Burn injury, application of clinically relevant continuum model to families with, **155–161**
    barriers and solutions for care of, 159–160
    family centered care, 156
    future research directions, 160–161
    sibling experiences, study of, 156–157
        findings, 157–158
    standards of care, 158–159
    use of evidence to provide care, 160

C

Cancer, views of rural providers and patients on screening for colorectal, **181–192**

Cardiovascular disease, translation of family health history questions for Latinas on, **207–218**

Nurs Clin N Am 46 (2011) 249–253
doi:10.1016/S0029-6465(11)00021-1
0029-6465/11/$ – see front matter © 2011 Elsevier Inc. All rights reserved.

nursing.theclinics.com

Moving?

Make sure your subscription moves with you!

To notify us of your new address, find your **Clinics Account Number** (located on your mailing label above your name), and contact customer service at:

Email: journalscustomerservice-usa@elsevier.com

800-654-2452 (subscribers in the U.S. & Canada)
314-447-8871 (subscribers outside of the U.S. & Canada)

Fax number: 314-447-8029

Elsevier Health Sciences Division
Subscription Customer Service
3251 Riverport Lane
Maryland Heights, MO 63043

*To ensure uninterrupted delivery of your subscription, please notify us at least 4 weeks in advance of move.

Printed and bound by CPI Group (UK) Ltd, Croydon, CR0 4YY

03/10/2024

01040456-0009